DIABETES and EXERCISE

OTHER BOOKS BY DR. ROBERT CANTU

Toward Fitness
Health Maintenance through Physical Conditioning
The Exercising Adult
Sports Medicine for the Primary Care Physician

*A Practical, Positive Way
to Control Diabetes*

DIABETES
and
EXERCISE

Dr. Robert C. Cantu, M.D., F.A.C.S.

With a Foreword by Thomas M. Flood, M.D.
Harvard University and the Joslin Diabetes Center

E. P. Dutton, Inc. · New York

Published in the United States by
E. P. Dutton, Inc.,
2 Park Avenue, New York, N.Y. 10016

Library of Congress Cataloging in Publication Data
Cantu, Robert C.
Diabetes and exercise.
Bibliography: p. 129
1. Exercise therapy.   2. Diabetes—Treatment.
I. Title.
RC661.E94C36   1981   616.4′62062   81-19463
                                       AACR2

ISBN: 0-525-93235-6 (cloth)
ISBN: 0-525-93236-4 (paper)

Published simultaneously in Canada by
Clarke, Irwin & Company Limited, Toronto and Vancouver

Designed by Nancy Scarino

10 9 8 7 6 5 4 3 2

First Edition

For Jane, Rob, and Biz

Contents

Acknowledgments

I would like to express my sincere appreciation to Dr. Thomas Flood of the Harvard Medical School and Joslin Clinic for his thoughtful foreword to this work. The same sentiments, and so much more, to my wife Jane Quale Cantu for inspiring this work and for sharing her insights and her life with me and our children. I also want to thank a talented writer and artist, Victor Wright Quale, for the illustrations in this book. I wish to acknowledge my appreciation to Human Sciences Press and especially Norma Fox, executive vice-president, for allowing me to use some of the material from *Toward Fitness* in this book, and to my secretary Pat Blackey, whose skills facilitated the preparation of this manuscript. Finally, I want to thank the editors at Dutton for their excellent assistance, which so cogently confirms the quote "No author is a genius to his publisher."

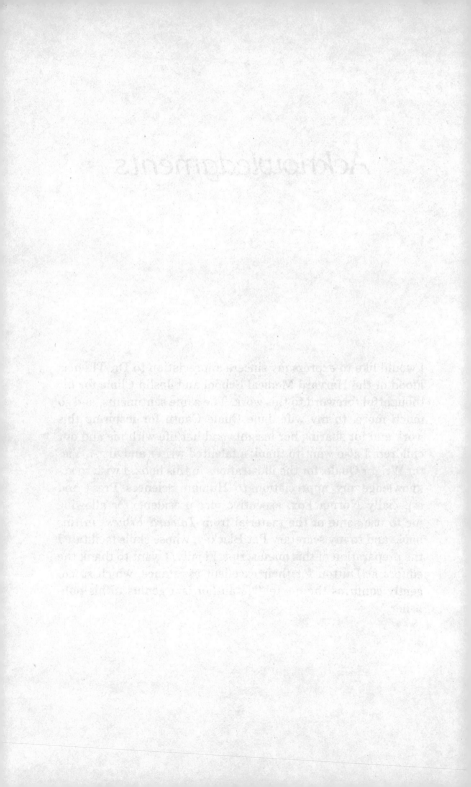

Foreword

The concept that exercise is beneficial to the diabetic is far from new: It was advocated as far back in antiquity as 600 A.D. by Chao Yuan-Fang, an eminent Chinese physician of the Sui Dynasty. Through the years, many noted specialists have recognized the value to the diabetic of regular physical activity and have encouraged their patients to exercise. However, they offered this advice sporadically and in an unspecific way. In sharp contrast to diet and insulin therapy, exercise as a treatment for diabetes was a half-forgotten and neglected stepchild.

Happily, a new era seems to have arrived. As we enter the decade of the eighties, a great surge of interest in physical fitness is occurring as a marvelous worldwide phenomenon. There is an increased recognition that individuals with diabetes mellitus can participate and derive benefits equal, in terms of enjoyment and improved good health, to those achieved by the nondiabetic. In addition, exercise, when integrated with a total diabetes treatment plan, offers unique advantages in terms of improved blood sugar regulation.

With *Diabetes and Exercise,* Dr. Robert Cantu has produced an excellent text and one that meets a real need. There is no shortage of exercise instruction manuals on the market. And there are a number of texts and guidebooks written to assist diabetics in the management of their disease. But now, for the first time, exercise and diabetes management are brought together in an easily understood, enjoyable format.

Those patients with insulin-dependent diabetes present the greatest challenge in terms of integrating an exercise program into the total plan of diabetes management. Because of individual differences, it is not possible to give absolutely specific advice, that is, to increase the diet by a certain amount or to decrease the insulin by so many units, and to expect this to work well in every case. Rather, one must deal with general principles and make adjustments based on symptoms and the results of test observations. Careful records of frequent urine or blood test results can be invaluable in fine-tuning the program to the individual. For example, most athletes do not perform well when hypoglycemic, and symptoms of low blood sugar during exercise clearly indicate a need for an increase in dietary carbohydrate or a reduction in insulin. On the other hand, the poorly controlled diabetic with marked elevation in blood sugar and acidic ketone bodies is not helped by exercise and may well deteriorate further, a situation that is certainly incompatible with deriving enjoyment or health benefit from physical activity.

In the May 1980 issue of the journal *Medical Times,* Dr. Fred W. Whitehouse, past president of the American Diabetes Association, stated, "It is clear that the healthiest diabetics are those who are trim and active." Dr. Cantu deserves the sincere thanks of diabetics and the medical community for the encouragement this text provides.

THOMAS M. FLOOD, M.D.,
Assistant Director of Education,
Joslin Diabetes Foundation

Boston, Massachusetts
September 9, 1980

Introduction

CAN DIET AND EXERCISE PREVENT DIABETES?

The answer to this question is an emphatic yes.

The incidence of diabetes in different societies of the same race may differ as much as ten times depending on environmental work and dietary circumstances. Diabetes is common in some groups of whites, blacks, Indians, native Americans, Chinese, Japanese, Polynesians, and Jews, whereas it is rare in other groups of the same ethnic background who eat less meat and saturated fat and expend more than 2,000 calories in exertion weekly. This suggests that in a majority of adult cases, diabetes can be prevented and that the major predisposing factors are excessive weight and inadequate exercise.

It is now quite evident that exercise is critical to the prevention and management of diabetes because, in addition to lowering blood sugar and keeping weight down, exercise seems to increase the longevity of some of the body's important cells.

In the past decade, concepts of diabetes mellitus have been in a state of evolution as new biologic characteristics of the disease have been exposed. Today, most diabetologists consider diabetes to be not one but several diseases, probably with multiple causes and mechanisms of transmission. But the cardinal feature is relative deficiency of the insulin-secreting (beta) cells of the pancreas, which produce carbohydrate intolerance—an inability to utilize carbohydrates. There are now more than 10 million diabetics in the United States, and the number is expected to exceed 20 million by the 1990s. If present trends continue, in the United States alone, one out of every five persons will contract this disease. Diabetes and the complications resulting from it are the third leading cause of death in the United States, following right behind cardiovascular disease and cancer. The direct and indirect effects of diabetes on the U.S. economy are staggering, exceeding $5 billion per year.

Before the discovery of insulin in 1921 by Sir Frederick Grant Banting and Charles Herbert Best, diabetes was fatal. Today, although not curable, it *is* largely controllable. The well regulated adult-onset (noninsulin-dependent) diabetic can anticipate a near-normal life expectancy. The outlook for the juvenile (insulin-dependent) diabetic is not quite as favorable owing to vascular complications that frequently occur after the disease has been present for several decades.

There have been many famous and accomplished people who were also diabetics: Nobel prize winner Dr. George R. Minot, who discovered the cause and treatment for pernicious anemia; H. G. Wells, the writer-historian; Giacomo Puccini, composer of the operas *La Bohème* and *Madama Butterfly;* French painter Paul Cezanne; and politician Fiorello LaGuardia. Actress Mary Tyler Moore is a diabetic, as are Jim "Catfish" Hunter of baseball, Bobby Clark of hockey, and tennis superstars Ham Richardson and the late Bill Tilden.

WHY A DIABETICS' EXERCISE BOOK?

"The ends must justify the means."
MATTHEW PRIOR (1664–1721)

Diabetes is a highly personal disease. All who have it, as well as their family members, know this. The medical profession, too, knows that, although exciting advances continue in research and treatment, in the last analysis it is still up to the diabetic patient to control his or her own health. This has been true since the discovery of insulin in 1921.

My personal involvement with the disease began in the fall of 1970, when my wife's diabetic condition was discovered. During my graduate work at the University of California, San Francisco, Medical Center, one of the areas I was particularly interested in was nutrition. I have always been a sports enthusiast. Today, as a neurosurgeon, fellow of the American College of Sports Medicine, and director of a Sports Medicine Service, I have rekindled those old interests. Since diabetes touched my home, I have been investigating the effects of nutrition and exercise on blood sugar and energy with a recharged personal interest.

Exercise has advantages specific to the diabetic. First, exercise increases the receptivity of muscle to insulin. Normally, a given amount of insulin will cause a certain amount of glucose to be picked up by a muscle cell. If that cell is exercised, the amount of glucose that is picked up is significantly increased. Thus, the same amount of insulin will allow increased amounts of glucose to be transferred from the bloodstream into the muscle.

Second, exercise helps by decreasing excess fat and increasing the body's cells sensitivity to insulin. Obesity itself reduces the sensitivity to insulin, therefore increasing a person's chances of acquiring diabetes and the complications from the disease. It is estimated that exercise and diet alone, by preventing obesity, can eliminate the occurrence of most adult-onset diabetes.

Third, exercise reduces the *triglycerides* and low density *lipoproteins* in the blood, which leads to better control of the diabetic state.* In addition to these advantages, which are unique to the diabetic, exercise also affords the diabetic the same (more than thirty) cardiovascular, pulmonary, circulatory, and emotional benefits that everybody else receives from exercise, such as feeling better, having a better outlook on life and oneself, and having more energy.

Having observed the benefits of exercise and diet in my wife's control of her diabetes, I have gone on to contact diabetic athletes in an attempt to establish some ground rules. I have included their stories and personal comments as they apply. Although marathon running is a remarkable achievement, most of these runners run only a marathon or two a year; the rest of the year their training is at a far more modest (20 to 30 miles per week) pace, which ensures the benefits of exercise without the risks of injury. It is my hope that other diabetics may gain insight and encouragement from their experiences and wish to take advantage of today's knowledge in the combined areas of diet, medication, and exercise to set new goals of fitness for themselves. From those who wish to compete in vigorous sports to those who desire only to "keep in shape," diabetics can all derive measurable advantages from a guided exercise program. For fit diabetics, the ends (good control without overinsulinizing) more than justify the means (discipline, energy, and regular exercise). That is why I have written this book: so that those who stand to gain the most from regular exertion will not be deterred, as they were in former times, because "they have diabetes."

---

* J. Wahren, L. Hagenfeldt, and P. Felig, "Glucose and free fatty acid utilization in exercise," *Israel Journal Medical Science* 11 (1975): 551–9.

DIABETES and EXERCISE

1.

The Triad: Diet, Insulin, and Exercise

THE DISEASE ITSELF

Diabetes is a condition characterized by a relative insulin deficiency resulting in an abnormal fuel-hormone response, especially when challenged by the ingestion of food. This abnormal fuel-hormone response involves a decreased storage and utilization of fuels and results in elevated blood levels of glucose (or sugar), free fatty acids, and ketones. Diabetes results from a deficiency in the insulin-secretory mechanism of the beta cells of the pancreas, a faulty insulin-receptor site on the cell surfaces of liver, adipose, and muscle tissue, and/or a metabolic defect in the cell itself.

There are two basic types of diabetes: insulin-dependent and noninsulin-dependent. As shown, insulin-dependent diabetics are usually under twenty years of age at the onset of disease. As a group they constitute less than 10 percent of the diabetic population. Their symptoms of diabetes are acute, coming speedily to a crisis: *Metabolic ketoacidosis* and insulin reactions are frequent, insulin production is decreased, the potential for developing maximal performance capacity is reduced, and hyperglycemia usually results from the marked reductions in glucose storage and utilization. Noninsulin-dependent diabetics, however, are generally over forty years of age at the onset of diabetes. More than 90 percent of all diabetics have this type of diabetes, and most have a family history of diabetes. The appearance of their symptoms is slow; they show a delayed insulin response to eating a meal, and hyperglycemia often results owing to the failure of the liver to retain glucose and to a small impairment in glucose oxidation.

TABLE 1
THE DIFFERENCES BETWEEN THE KINDS OF DIABETES

	INSULIN-DEPENDENT	NONINSULIN-DEPENDENT
Age at onset	Usually under 20	Usually over 40
Proportion of all diabetics	Less than 10 percent	Greater than 90 percent
Appearance of symptoms	Acute or subacute	Slow
Metabolic ketoacidosis	Frequent	Rare
Obesity at onset	Uncommon	Common
Beta cells	Decreased	Variable
Insulin	Decreased	Variable
Family history of diabetes	Uncommon	Common

THE FOOD AND INSULIN BALANCE

Insulin-dependent diabetes treatment requires insulin replacement therapy, which must be appropriately balanced with the dietary intake and energy expenditure. The goal of treatment is to normalize the storage and utilization of metabolic fuels by attempting to keep blood glucose as close to normal as possible. Recently improved management programs involve the use of various insulins that act at different times throughout the day. (See Figure 1.) In general, insulin-dependent diabetics will take a combination of quick-acting insulin, which peaks in two to three hours, and an intermediate-acting insulin, which peaks in seven to eight hours but has a lasting effect over the whole day. Many may take multiple insulin injections; the most common is the split dose, or about two-thirds of the daily dosage in the morning and the other one-third before supper or at bedtime.

The noninsulin-dependent diabetic exhibits a delayed rise in insulin secretion in response to eating. In other words, instead of reaching a peak insulin secretion in response to a carbohydrate meal in one hour, the response is delayed until two hours. This type of diabetic also has less liver retention of glucose; this leads to increased blood sugar in the circulation after a meal and a somewhat lower than normal rate of utilization of glucose by muscle and adipose tissue. A majority are overweight or obese and have a low oxidation rate for carbohydrate, which is believed to be because the interaction of insulin at the cell surface or within the cell itself has been reduced. Aerobic exercise can enhance this vital interaction of insulin at the cellular level.

Inadequate physical activity and excessive caloric intake are the two most important environmental factors influencing the development of diabetes. Endurance exercise programs have great potential for the restoration of normal metabolism, since both a loss of weight and endurance training enhance the action of insulin, that is, make it more potent. Moderate sustained activity will result in a gradual reduction in blood glucose (sugar) as the exercising muscle takes up and utilizes that glucose for energy. This decrease will frequently last for one or more days after the exercise ceases. Endurance exercise also increases cellular sensitivity to insulin, thus the same amount

3

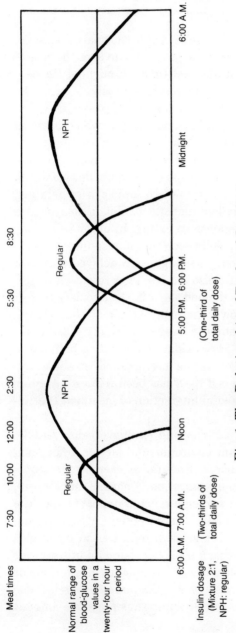

Meal times

7:30 10:00 12:00 2:30 5:30 8:30 Midnight 6:00 A.M.

6:00 A.M. 7:00 A.M.   Noon   5:00 P.M. 6:00 P.M.

Normal range of blood-glucose values in a twenty-four hour period

Regular   NPH   Regular   NPH

Insulin dosage
(Mixture 2:1,
NPH: regular)

(Two-thirds of
total daily dose)

(One-third of
total daily dose)

Fig. 1. The Relationship of Food and Insulin*

The insulin-dependent patient's daily food is given as three meals and three between-meal snacks (the most common and desirable pattern of food intake for nondiabetic children). Insulin is given in two daily doses of a 2:1 mixture of NPH: regular, two-thirds of the dosage in the morning and the remaining one-third in the afternoon.

Regular insulin takes effect quickly and lasts for only four to six hours. NPH insulin, on the other hand, lasts for about twelve to fourteen hours. Thus, the regimen maintains blood glucose levels as close to normal as possible for the diabetic child throughout a twenty-four hour period, and it helps prevent both urinary spilling of glucose and hypoglycemia.

* From Robert L. Jackson and Richard Guthrie, Current Concepts®: *The Child with Diabetes Mellitus*, Kalamazoo: The Upjohn Co., 1975.

of insulin will allow the cell to utilize an increased amount of sugar.

The use of exercise in the treatment of diabetes is certainly not new: It was recommended therapy for the disease in India as early as 600 B.C. Dr. Elliott P. Joslin of Boston, a world-renowned diabetologist, was a staunch advocate of exercise prior and subsequent to the discovery of insulin in 1921. He stressed that optimal treatment of diabetes consists of a triad balancing the insulin dose and dietary intake with exercise. Today, this course still appears to be the most sensible and effective one.

In prescribing exercise for the diabetic patient, two distinct programs must be established. First, all diabetics must be evaluated and assigned to an exercise program based upon whether or not they have vascular complications. The diabetic is twenty-five times more susceptible to blindness, seventeen times more susceptible to kidney disease, five times more susceptible to gangrene and amputation, and twice as prone to heart disease than the nondiabetic, all because of vulnerability to vascular disease. Those patients who have been screened and who are *without* vascular complications may be assigned to a regular adult fitness program. Patients *with* vascular complications—eye (*retinopathy*), kidney (*nephropathy*), coronary heart disease, or peripheral vascular disease—should follow a cardiac rehabilitation program until they reach the minimum fitness and endurance level necessary for inclusion into a regular adult fitness program. The identification of vascular complications must be made by the patient's personal physician, and his permission for participation in such a rehabilitation program must be obtained.

Is there one basic diabetic exercise program? The answer, of course, is no. An exercise prescription should be written in the very same manner as it would be for any nondiabetic adult once the initial screening has been successfully completed. It is

5

still essential, however, to realize that *optimal control of diabetes at any stage is possible only with optimal dietary control.*

But physicians themselves, accustomed to prescribing medicines, are sometimes guilty of using insulin too liberally and of not selling diet and exercise enthusiastically and forcefully enough. More than 90 percent of adult-onset diabetics are above ideal body weight. It is well known that the incidence of obesity increases with age, as does the incidence of diabetes. Nine in ten cases of adult-onset diabetes are triggered by excessive caloric intake and resultant obesity.*

Diet and exercise alone, with a reduction and then maintenance of body weight at ideal levels, will eliminate the diabetes. *To reiterate, 90 percent of adult-onset diabetes is preventable with a proper dietary-exercise regimen.*† I feel strongly that a newly detected adult diabetic should not start any medication until a faithfully executed dietary-exercise program has been thoroughly tried. As Dr. Tom Flood of the Joslin Diabetes Foundation in Boston states, "One should give diet and exercise a trial of at least a month before weighing alternatives. The aim is to attain a rather sharp drop in weight, to 'reset' the insulin receptors, and demonstrate to the patient that diet alone is effective and specific therapy."

Diabinese and Tolbutamide are oral hypoglycemic agents that augment insulin secretion by the beta cells of the pancreas. They are inadvisable in juvenile-onset diabetes, severe or unstable diabetes, and diabetes complicated by ketoacidosis, infection, trauma, pregnancy, or by kidney, thyroid, or liver disease. Until recently, they had been used in many adult-onset diabetics. Recent studies have suggested they may be associated with an increased risk of heart attack; thus, today, their use is very limited. It is probable that there was increased risk of heart attack because many who used these agents did so

---

* K. Gabbay, "New Directions in Diabetes," *Children's World* 4 (1977): 2–17.
† K. M. West and J. M. Kalbfleisch, "Influence of Nutritional Factors on Prevalence of Diabetes," *Diabetes* 20 (1971): 99–108.

while neglecting diet and exercise and, as a result, had elevated blood-sugar levels. Today we stress diet and exercise and, for the 10 percent not controlled by this regimen, appropriate supplemental insulin.

But all too frequently, diabetic training programs tend to overstress the role of insulin in diabetes control. Teaching emphasizes the potency of the insulin substance, the need for precise measurement, and the proper injection technique. The need for proper eating is often not given the same emphasis, and the patient thinks it has secondary importance. The result: He is extremely cautious with insulin and quite incautious with eating. Obviously, it is much easier for both the physician and the patient to increase insulin rather than to come to grips with proper dietary and exercise management. For the doctor, it takes less time to prescribe a few more units of insulin, than it does to sell a dietary and exercise plan and to check and recheck that the patient is faithfully adhering to it.

The objective, then, is to set up a complementary program of diet and exercise! But I will be the first to admit that a regular regimen of both is not an easy accomplishment. It *does* require some alteration of life-style. Undoubtedly, this explains why so many physicians will not even prescribe specific diet and exercise programs for their diabetic patients. They have experienced so much failure in other areas of patient care that attempt to change life patterns—even in simple assignments like diet plans—that the idea of expecting a diabetic to follow a demanding total conditioning program for the rest of his or her life seems difficult.

Still, I am confident that most diabetics after reading this book will be convinced of the absolute value of exercise to their health and will undertake and maintain a regular conditioning program. And they will need to make only minimal sacrifices, since the exercise program outlined in this book is designed to permit individuals to write their own exercise prescriptions based on physical activities that they normally perform and enjoy both at work and play. Finally, while the nondiabetic may skip a set of tennis because he feels guilty about "having fun" instead of working, diabetics should realize that exercise is vital to their daily medical treatment and that only by pursuing it can they be at their best.

2.

Diet

SOME DANGEROUS PATTERNS

Consider the Japanese sumo wrestlers. They are massively overweight to the point of being bulbous. They must overeat continually to maintain their size, which is important partly to enable them to pin and throw their opponents and partly for style. In this traditional Japanese sport, the public expects its heroes to be *very* fat.

So sumo wrestlers consume food high in starch. Individuals recruited to this profession because of their size are placed immediately on diets containing up to 6,000 calories, 80 percent of it carbohydrate. While they are in training for their sport, sumo wrestlers exercise intensely but over short periods of time, not in a manner that would develop the cardiovascular endurance that physiologists consider essential for good health. During this "training" they continually gain weight.

They also develop diabetes.

The incidence of diabetes among Japanese sumo wrestlers is extremely high, particularly when compared with the average man on the street. One study showed that 60 percent of the wrestlers had glucose-tolerance curves considered "diabetic." This compared with a level of only 5 percent for the normal Japanese population. Ten percent of the wrestlers needed insulin treatment as opposed to 1 percent of the normal population. In addition, 25 percent suffered from diabetic retinopathy, the side effect of the disease that severely affects vision and may eventually cause blindness.

While achieving fame in the ring, these sumo wrestlers obviously were destroying their health. Equally obvious is the relationship of obesity and overeating to diabetes. The wrestlers overate themselves into a diabetic state. This is true not merely among sumo wrestlers but also among the general population.

More than 90 percent of adult-onset noninsulin-dependent diabetics are overweight. It is a fact that if you overeat, you may not necessarily contract diabetes, but you certainly increase your chances of doing so. If you have a diabetic condition, you may complicate that condition by continuing to overeat. The reverse of that equation, however, is that if you can control your diet, you may be able to control your diabetic condition.

Diabetes generally is considered to be an inherited disease. If you are a diabetic, particularly a juvenile-onset insulin-dependent diabetic, there is an increased chance that your children may become diabetic, simply because of their similar genetic makeup. But your diabetic condition also may be partly a result of your life-style, if that life-style causes you to be overweight.

There are 10 million diabetics in America, 8.5 million of them classified as adult-onset diabetics. Of this group, 90 percent (or 7.65 million) are overweight. These overweight diabetics can control their diabetes condition and sometimes *eliminate* it by using diet and exercise to maintain a proper body weight.

What does this mean concerning the total number of diabetics of all types? Simply that of the 10 million American diabetics, 7.65 million of them (or three out of every four individuals) could prevent the disease! In the light of this information, the fact that diabetes should remain so widespread seems astounding.

Moreover, if most cases of diabetics can be prevented through diet and exercise, why is the number of diabetics increasing? One reason is that many people are careless and lazy about their health. Or they have not been warned properly about the danger of overeating coupled with physical inactivity. Or if warned, they have ignored the warning. Certainly people continue to smoke despite the well-advertised connection between smoking and lung cancer.

As people get older, the incidence of obesity increases. This is as much a matter of reduced activity and reduced metabolism as it is of increased food intake. The incidence of diabetes also increases with age.

The incidence of diabetes among different societies of the same race may differ as much as ten times depending on environmental, work, and dietary circumstances.

Diabetes is common in certain groups of whites, blacks, Indians, Native Americans, Chinese, Japanese, Polynesians, and Jews, yet rare in other groups of the same ethnic background who eat and exercise differently. This suggests that in a majority of adult cases, diabetes is preventable and that the major predisposing factors are a high-caloric diet and inadequate exercise. Without question, the risk of diabetes is greatly enhanced by excessive caloric intake, whether the calories come from fat, protein, or carbohydrate.

So the overweight person who is identified as a diabetic should reduce. In fact, weight reduction through diet should be the first treatment that a physician recommends.

If weight loss is required, the overweight diabetic may need to limit dietary intake to no more than 1,000 to 1,500 calories a day. Such a diet should provide weight loss of approximately two pounds per week. If the diet is as low as 1,000 calories, it should be balanced evenly over the day and chosen with the aid of a dietician. Addition of a daily multivitamin supplement may be necessary, but vitamin pills are not substitutes for proper nutrition and excessive use of them should be avoided.

Although 1,000 calories a day may cause a person used to generous helpings to think he is hardly eating at all, he will not starve. Dolly Cmiel, a registered dietician, explains: "Most people will be surprised by the different types of foods they are allowed to eat on a low-calorie diet. The most important fact is not the quality but the quantity of foods to be consumed." (Examples of low-calorie menus are presented in appendix II.)

The major problem that diabetic dieters will face when they begin their weight-reducing diets is hunger. However, the overt symptoms of diabetes—excessive thirst (polydipsia) and excessive urination (polyuria)—will abate.

Even for the insulin-dependent diabetic, diet remains the most important means of achieving good control without insulin reactions. Only when this fact is not adequately stressed in the orientation of a new diabetic patient or when the patient ignores the dietary advice offered do problems occur. Control may be very difficult to obtain in certain conditions. If the diabetic is an alcoholic or a compulsive eater, physician and patient may be wasting their time. A person who is chronically inebriated will not possess the mental discipline necessary for dietary management. The same is true with a compulsive eater, for whom food provides a form of drunkenness. The physician who focuses on the diabetes in such cases may be treating the wrong disease. If the person is unwilling or unable to change his drinking or eating habits to conform to the requirements of the prescribed diet, psychiatric help may be necessary.

Sheer boredom is another adversary of dietary control. Education leading to an increased knowledge about foods and their preparation can help a diabetic improve his diet. Those responsible for promoting better diabetic nutrition need to learn that they must do more than merely hand a diabetic a dietary sheet with instructions to "follow these guidelines." They need to teach him to understand the basics of nutrition and how to utilize the exchange lists in creating both a safe and appetizing diet.

Many diabetics become gourmet chefs in their own kitchens. Those who fail to take an interest in their own feeding may condemn themselves to a life of culinary mediocrity with its risks of dietary indiscretion, inappropriate calorie intake, and poor control. Eating out presents another problem for the diabetic. The nondiabetic visits restaurants seeking gourmet dishes. But the diabetic handed an oversized menu with its fancy names, fancy printing, and fancy prices must read it with some trepidation, since the precise nutrient and caloric content of the food on it is most likely unavailable. It is a good idea to have the waiter or waitress help you choose the foods right for your diet. Strange dishes probably ought to be avoided. When eating out diabetics must stick to plain, wholesome dishes and eat amounts of each food according to their own dietary plan. Only at home, where they can be certain of the precise ingredients of what they eat, can diabetics treat themselves to true gourmet dishes.

What can the diabetic expect when he changes his diet? Improved health may be the major result. Many physicians are finally becoming aware that a diet program, particularly if it is coupled with exercise, can prevent many of the vascular complications often associated with diabetes. It is a fact that individuals with normal blood-sugar levels simply do not suffer the injuries to the blood vessels associated with diabetes, namely retinopathy of the eye and glomerulosclerosis of the kidney. Studies show this to be true throughout the world.

This raises an interesting point: If these injuries to the vessels were caused only by a genetic defect unrelated to hyperglycemia (high blood sugar), then we might expect to encounter them in at least some individuals whose blood-sugar levels were not high. Since these problems appear only in hyperglycemic individuals (that is, diabetics), it tells us that by preventing or limiting high blood sugar alone, we can limit these dangerous side effects.

And the best way to lower blood sugar? Diet and exercise, of course.

Additional studies also indicate that diet influences the rate of coronary disease. This is true of the general population, but it is particularly true with diabetics. Put in its most blunt terms, the North American high-fat and high-calorie diet is a killer.

Consider these statistics. Diabetic coronary disease appears two to ten times more frequently in North America than in certain Asian, African, and Latin American societies. The dissimilarity cannot be attributed to genetic or racial differences, since statistics related to people of different ethnic stock shift as they shift continents. Coronary disease is several times higher among diabetic black Americans than among diabetic Nigerians. Death from cardiovascular complications occurs much less frequently among diabetic men and women living in Japan than among those of Japanese descent living in Hawaii. These differences are due primarily to variations in diet and work habits. In a comparison of diabetic men and women of Japanese ancestry on the island of Hawaii and in Hiroshima, the caloric intake was roughly equal, but the daily consumption of fat was twice as high in the Hawaiian Japanese. Furthermore, the Hawaiian Japanese ate predominantly saturated fats. In these two groups, the incidence of diabetes was not significantly different. However, the incidence of elevated blood cholesterol and triglyceride levels (which coincide statistically with elevated coronary death rates) was much higher in the Hawaiian Japanese, even among people who were not obese. And it was true among nonobese Hawaiians compared to obese Hiroshimans. Moreover, the number of vascular complications of diabetes causing death, especially heart attack, was twice as great in the Hawaiian Japanese. Their mortality rate mimicked the Hawaiian white population whose life-style they shared.

The vascular complications in diabetes are influenced by the amount of saturated fat in the diet and resultant blood cholesterol levels. The basic reason that fat is so harmful for those controlling their weight is because every ounce of fat has more than twice as many calories as every ounce of protein or carbohydrate. Saturated fat intake may be a greater risk factor for heart attack than diabetes itself. It certainly suggests that a reduction in fat intake for subjects with diabetes may be the most important approach to prevention of *ischemic heart disease*.

Overweight diabetics should also obviously decrease their number of calories, decrease the frequency of feedings (fewer between-meal snacks), and not use food to treat high blood sugar. These rules do not necessarily apply to the nonobese diabetic, the person who does not have trouble maintaining his weight. The nonobese diabetic, however, should maintain daily consistency of calorie consumption and be consistent about when he eats. If this person exercises, as we recommend, he may need to allow for extra food intake, whereas the obese diabetic cannot afford this luxury.

A PERSONAL BALANCE

As long as *diabetics* control their balance of calories consumed and calories burned, they can tolerate diets high in carbohydrates. This runs counter to some previous dietary principles that held that a diabetic diet should be high in protein and high in fat. Diabetics still need to curtail their intake of simple carbohydrates, such as refined sugar, honey, syrups, and jellies, but they can consume the complex carbohydrates found in pasta and vegetables without fear as long as they do not exceed their caloric limits. Individuals who exercise will find that their bodies will demand more complex carbohydrates in their diets. One other point: In general, diabetics should reduce the saturated-fat levels in their diets to about half the traditional level. This energy source can be replaced with unsaturated vegetable fat or starch.

As is true for nondiabetics, the rate of coronary disease for diabetics is influenced by blood cholesterol levels. Diets high in saturated fat result in high blood cholesterol levels—what is known in the medical literature as hypercholesterolemia. To a lesser extent, high blood sugar also seems to produce hypercholesterolemia. Serum cholesterol is highest in those diabetics in poor control. Thus, when we begin to decide what diet to prescribe for a diabetic, we should limit not only calorie intake, but also saturated fat. Fatty meats, egg yolks, butter, and other whole milk dairy products may prove even more harmful to the diabetic than they are to the nondiabetic.

Each diabetic diet should be tailored to the individual. In addition, the needs of the insulin-dependent diabetic vary substantially from those of the noninsulin-dependent, obese, adult-onset diabetic. One major difference is that the overweight diabetic should attempt to improve the pancreatic beta-cell function. When a person is overweight, his muscle cells may lose their sensitivity to insulin. It requires more insulin to cause the cells to absorb the glucose in the bloodstream. With the overweight diabetic, it often is not a matter that the body produces *less* insulin but rather that the body now needs *more* insulin for proper glycogen storage. An overweight person, thus, is often considered out of balance in more ways than one. But the condition is reversible. Reducing weight results in a similar reduction of the relative amount of insulin needed, with the bottom line being that the formerly obese person can no longer be classified as a diabetic. Japanese sumo wrestlers can eliminate their diabetic condition by avoiding the excessive dietary regimen that caused them to gain weight. They will lose their wrestling jobs, but they will preserve their health.

HOW TO PLAN YOUR INDIVIDUAL DIET

The diabetic diet is merely a modification of the diet that *every* person needs to maintain health. It is essential for the diabetic to find a diet that best fits his or her individual needs. Most doctors use a food exchange system to prescribe diets for their patients, and this system provides a relatively easy way for the diabetic to plan meals and maintain good control. You must understand that the exchange system is not the diabetic diet; it is merely a tool that most people working with diabetics find makes meal planning easier.

The system of food exchanges affords the diabetic flexibility in choice of foods while maintaining consistency of total calories and diet composition. The insulin-dependent diabetic who acquires a knowledge of diet can obtain flexibility in food choice even beyond the standard exchange lists. The noninsulin-dependent diabetic may not need to use exchange lists as long as that person avoids foods high in refined sugar or saturated fat while at the same time reducing total caloric intake.

The four principles of the diabetic diet are

1. Regulation of calories
2. Timing of meals
3. Regularity of meals
4. Individualizing the diet

The traditional meals that Americans eat are a small breakfast, a medium-sized lunch, and a heavy dinner. This is not the best meal plan for the diabetic. The diabetic should eat his meals at regular times during the day and should have approximately the same-sized meals. It is also best—and the diabetic diet is no exception—to eat the foods that you like, that you know how to prepare, and that you feel comfortable with. But you must modify these foods within the whole meal plan to meet the specific needs of your diabetic condition.

Each diabetic diet must be tailored to the individual. In addition, the needs of the insulin-dependent diabetic differ from those of the noninsulin-dependent, obese, adult-onset diabetic. The table below outlines some of the major differences.

TABLE 2
DIETARY PLAN FOR THE INSULIN-
AND NONINSULIN-DEPENDENT DIABETIC

PLAN	NONINSULIN-DEPENDENT DIABETIC		INSULIN-DEPENDENT DIABETIC	
	Nonobese	Obese	Nonobese	Obese
Decrease calories	No	Yes	No	Yes
Protect or improve pancreatic beta-cell function	Yes	Yes	No (beta cells usually extinct)	No
Increase frequency of feedings	No	No	Yes	Yes
Maintain consistent daily caloric, carbohydrate, protein and fat consumption	Yes	No (with low caloric consumption)	Yes	Yes
Time meals consistently	No	No	Yes	Yes
Allow extra food for unusual exercise	Yes	No	Yes (or reduce insulin injection)	Yes
Use food to treat or abort hypoglycemia	Yes	No	Yes	Yes

What is the exchange system? Exchange means that a food may be substituted for another food in a diet plan. The diet exchange system was devised to render meal planning simpler and yet more interesting, while at the same time ensuring that you consume not only the correct number of calories but also the proper amounts of protein, fats, and carbohydrates. For each meal, there is a menu based on the total daily calorie allotment with a prescribed amount of protein, carbohydrates, and fats. The actual foods themselves are listed in terms of "exchanges" as enumerated under six exchange lists: *milk, vegetables, fruit, bread, meat, fat.* Learning to use the exchange lists, however, takes some practice.

Normally when a person is diagnosed as diabetic, the doctor prescribes a diet limiting the amount of calories the person eats each day and dictating from which food types (exchanges) those calories should come. Each exchange within a group has approximately the same amount of calories, and there is a direct relationship between the exchange and number of calories. For instance, a typical 1,000-calorie diet would consist of about 15 exchanges, a 1,200-calorie diet might have around 18, and a 1,500-calorie diet 21. A person on a 1,500-calorie diet might eat for breakfast:

1 fruit exchange
2 bread exchanges
1 meat exchange
1 milk exchange
2 fat exchanges
coffee or tea

The 1,500-calorie plan for lunch

2 meat exchanges
2 bread exchanges
vegetables as desired

1 fruit exchange
1 milk exchange
1 fat exchange
coffee or tea

And, still, at the same level, the exchange list for dinner:

2 meat exchanges
1½ bread exchanges
1 vegetable exchange
1 fruit exchange
½ milk exchange
1 fat exchange
coffee or tea

The first time a diabetic confronts such an exchange list, it may appear confusing. Perhaps it would be easier, if instead of the word *exchange,* you thought instead of the word *portion.* In the fruit exchange list, one portion is one small apple, so two exchanges would be two small apples. Or twenty large cherries. Eventually, as you use the exchange list, it becomes simpler.

For example, the lunch menu above calls for two meat exchanges, so (consulting the lists that follow) you may decide to have two ounces of poultry or fish. Or you might elect to choose ¼ cup of cottage cheese and an egg. The menu also calls for two bread exchanges, therefore you can have two plain rolls. Or if you prefer, a cup of cooked rice or spaghetti.

It is important to understand that the foods given in any exchange are entirely your choice, but the amounts are not. Therefore, you must measure carefully. Also, consult your doctor regarding between-meal and nighttime snacks. Many diabetologists favor dividing the caloric consumption into three main meals and two or three snacks. Generally, they allot breakfast one-fifth of the daily caloric intake and the noon meal and dinner each two-fifths. The afternoon snack is sub-tracted from the noon meal and evening snack from dinner. Each snack should supply 10 to 15 grams of carbohydrate. If you desire a midmorning snack, subtract it from breakfast.

Appendix II lists six diabetic exchange lists to help you in planning your meals.

While the specific diet your doctor prescribes in terms of content and calories will be determined by your size and energy expenditure, certain general principles apply. Eat only the number of meals and amounts of foods as listed on your meal plan. Do not skip any meals, as this is asking for an insulin reaction. Take no medicine except that prescribed by your doctor. This is true for anyone, of course, but it is of special importance for the diabetic. Try to avoid specially packaged or dietetic candies and cakes unless you first ask your doctor or dietician.

Many seasonings, such as spices, herbs, and salt, may be used in unlimited amounts and at any time without measuring. Foods and beverages, such as coffee and tea, fat-free broth, unsweetened gelatin, and sour or dill pickles, can also be consumed without limit. Foods that generally are to be avoided unless permitted by your doctor are sugar, candy, jelly, marmalade, cakes, regular soft drinks, alcoholic beverages, fried foods, and syrups.

To show how this food exchange system works, let us look at a low-calorie (1,500 a day) diet breakfast. It is recommended to eat 1 fruit, 2 breads, 1 meat, 2 fats, and 1 milk exchange. With these restrictions, you could have ½ cup of orange juice, ½ cup of cooked cereal, 1 slice of toast with a teaspoon of butter, 1 egg, 1 slice of bacon, and 1 cup of milk. Not as bad a breakfast as you might expect!

What happens if you decide to go out to Long John Silver's for some fish and chips? A low-calorie diet person would limit his intake, but the nonobese diabetic may not have to. If he ordered a two-piece dinner of fish, chips, and coleslaw, the diabetic could count this as 6 bread, 4 meat, and 6 fat exchanges.

This meal could be easily handled by a diabetic on an effective diet and exercise program.

There has been much controversy over the use of saccharin in our foods. It is believed to be related to an increased incidence of bladder cancer. The Diabetes Association fought to keep saccharin on the grocery shelves because they felt that a ban would cause problems for diabetics who were not able to use other kinds of sweeteners. They felt that not being able to use saccharin would create more problems for the diabetic than the slight increased risk of cancer.

Alcohol also has been questioned much for its use by diabetics. You must remember that alcohol does add calories, just as any other food or drink. It is possible that alcohol can be used on a limited basis, but the individual should get a doctor's opinion on this matter.

Often diabetics will question the use of fructose in their diet. It is a corn sweetener that is metabolized a little differently from, and more efficiently than, sucrose. For this reason, it is thought to be more acceptable for the diabetic person.

If the diabetic complies with his diet prescription and food exchanges, control through diet therapy is very feasible. This is especially true for the most common type of diabetes—adult diabetes in the overweight person. Diet therapy, especially in conjunction with an exercise program, not only will control the disease but also may reverse it in many individuals. *It has been estimated that half of all diabetics in the United States and other affluent societies could be "cured" by reversal of obesity to optimal body weight and subsequent regulation of caloric intake to match caloric expenditure.* In the lean, insulin-dependent diabetic, diet therapy rarely "cures" the disease, but in conjunction with exercise, regulation is enhanced and vascular complications are lessened.

In 1973 Professor Victor Herbert, a medical scientist, stated unequivocally that the sole indication of vitamin therapy is vitamin deficiency.* Elsewhere, it has been said that of the $160 million spent annually in this country on vitamin preparations, $140 million produces nothing but expensive urine! The American Medical Association has reported that "the use of multivitamin preparations as a form of dietary insurance is a common practice, but it is a poor practice. There is little harm so long as the preparations are not used to excess and the practice is not taken as justification for dietary lunacy." Obviously, a vitamin prescription may be called for in persons who through ignorance, poor eating habits, or emotional illness have deficient diets. And they may also be indicated for special periods of nutrient demand, such as during pregnancy, breast-feeding, or prolonged illness. They are also suggested for the overweight diabetic on a daily diet of 1,000 calories or less. However, for the stable diabetic, the need for supplemental vitamins is rare, since, like the vegetarian, he or she must be diet conscious.

While supplementary vitamins may help children and adults with inadequate diets, it should be realized that months of deprivation are required to deplete the body's store of fat-soluble vitamins. A few days of inadequate intake will not precipitate any health crises, except in the mind. Thus, when taking vitamins, follow the recommendation of the American Medical Association and use them only in specific instances of need. Remember that specific vitamins in therapeutic amounts should be prescribed only in the presence of vitamin deficiencies or increased requirements.

Menus for people with diabetes are also appropriate for other members of the family. In fact, your low-sugar, low-fat meal plan would probably be better for your friends and family than the diet they are currently eating. Also, you do not have to prepare special foods, as many nondiabetics think. Menus do not have to be complicated. Though it is not recommended,

* A. P. Fletch, "The Effect of Weight Reduction upon the Blood Pressure of Obese Hypertensives," *Quarterly Journal Medicine* 23 (1954): 331–45.

using the same menu for breakfast every morning is certainly acceptable. (Eating a variety of foods is a better guarantee for including all nutrients in your diet.) The important element is that you develop a system of meal preparation that will allow you to stick to the prescribed meal plan.

For those who like a variety of foods, a cookbook with recipes that give diabetic exchange values will be helpful. A word of caution, however—the exchange lists were changed in 1977. Be sure to use a cookbook that uses the same exchange values that are in your meal plan. By using the exchange lists, you can figure the values of your favorite recipes. When calculating these values, it may be easier to change the recipe slightly to meet exchange values than to deal in fractions of exchanges more complicated than one-fourth.

Almost always your prescribed diet will include a snack. Usually the snack contains about one-tenth of the day's total calories and, like the meals, offers a variety of foods. You will notice that the snack in our meal plan is limited to foods from the fruit and bread exchanges. Since drinking milk and eating foods with fat in them just before exercise sometimes causes nausea and cramping, we do not include these foods as suggested snacks. We arranged a sample meal plan to meet the needs of a person who engages in mild exercise (jogging a mile or two a day). Most people do not like to exercise after a meal, but the diabetic should not exercise when it has been several hours since he last ate. (Exercise increases the need for glucose.) It is suggested that the diabetic have a snack before and/or after exercise. Sample meal plans and recipes are presented in appendix II.

3.

The Metabolism of Insulin Use and Exercise

EXERCISE AND INSULIN

The beneficial effects of endurance training on the normal middle-aged heart include a slowing of the heart rate (brady-cardia), prolongation of *diastole* and thus increased blood flow to the heart muscle, increase in stroke volume and thus more efficient and powerful work of the heart muscle, reduced blood pressure, reduced clotting time and viscosity, or stickiness, of the blood, and a decrease in blood fats and their deposition in the body's blood vessels. These physiological changes in response to exercise occur in the diabetic and nondiabetic alike. However, since the diabetic is twice as prone to heart attack as the nondiabetic, these benefits of exercise take on added importance. As additional positive effects, endurance training for the diabetic and nondiabetic will:

BLOOD VESSELS AND CHEMISTRY

Increase blood oxygen content
Increase blood-cell mass and blood volume

25

Increase fibrinolytic capability

Increase efficiency of peripheral blood distribution and return

Increase blood supply to muscles and more efficient exchange of oxygen and carbon dioxide

Reduce serum triglycerides and cholesterol levels

Reduce platelet cohesion or stickiness

Reduce systolic and diastolic blood pressure, especially when elevated

Reduce glucose intolerance

HEART

Increase strength of cardiac contraction (myocardial efficiency)

Increase blood supply (collateral) to heart

Increase size of coronary arteries

Increase size of heart muscle

Increase blood volume (stroke volume) per heartbeat

Increase heart rate recovery after exercise

Reduce heart rate at rest

Reduce heart rate with exertion

Reduce vulnerability to cardiac arrhythmias

LUNGS

Increase blood supply

Increase diffusion of O_2 and CO_2

Increase functional capacity during exercise

Reduce nonfunctional volume of lung

ENDOCRINE (GLANDULAR) AND METABOLIC FUNCTION

Increase tolerance to stress

Increase glucose tolerance

Increase thyroid function
Increase growth hormone production
Increase lean muscle mass
Increase enzymatic function in muscle cells
Increase functional capacity during exercise (muscle oxygen uptake capacity)
Reduce body fat content
Reduce chronic catecholamine production
Reduce neurohumoral overreaction

NEURAL AND PSYCHIC

Reduce strain and nervous tension resulting from psychological stress
Reduce tendency for depression
Induce *joie de vivre*

Insulin enables the body's tissues to use glucose, the sole fuel for our brain. It makes possible the storage of glucose in our muscles and liver. The presence of insulin also retards the burning of body fat. Glucose is the preferred fuel for the cells of our body, and insulin is the hormone that allows cells to take glucose from the blood and burn (metabolize) it. When there is insufficient insulin, as in the insulin-dependent diabetic, the situation is analogous to starvation in the nondiabetic. Free fatty acids would be released from our fat stores to serve as a fuel source for our body's cells. Even protein or the muscle mass of our body is converted to a fuel source.

Following the discovery of insulin by Dr. Frederick Grant Banting and Dr. Charles Herbert Best in 1921, the beneficial effects of exercise continued to be emphasized by Joslin, who popularized the diet-exercise-insulin triad of diabetes treatment. It has long been recognized that insulin requirements decrease, often as much as 50 percent, when the diabetic undertakes a regular daily regimen of thirty to sixty minutes of vigorous physical activity, while carbohydrate intake may increase. In fact, in many adult-onset diabetics, exercise so improves glucose tolerance that insulin may no longer be required. To understand how exercise can accomplish this, we must first examine the metabolism of exercise in nondiabetics.

HOW EXERCISE WORKS

While fat and carbohydrates each contribute only about 40 percent to the caloric content of the average diet, the body stores fuel almost entirely (80 percent to 85 percent) in the form of fat, or triglycerides. The remainder of our immediate fuel source is glucose or sugar, which when stored in our muscles and the liver is called glycogen. During the earliest phase of muscular activity, the first five to ten minutes, it is the glycogen, the glucose stored in the muscles, that is the major fuel source. As exercise continues, glucose release from the liver increases and muscle blood flow and glucose uptake can rise seven to twenty times the resting level depending on the intensity of the exercise performed. As the duration and intensity of exercise increases, the liver continues to release glucose, both from its glycogen stores and by a process of making glucose from its simpler building blocks (lactate, pyruvate, glycerol, amino acids). The diabetic's liver, both at rest and while exercising, has an enhanced ability to synthesize or manufacture glucose.

In prolonged exercise (between one and four hours), the blood glucose level progressively falls and the level of stored fat, or triglycerides, released from adipose tissue rises and becomes the major fuel source. This slight fall in blood glucose level occurs because the liver is unable to keep pace with the muscles' continuing greatly increased demand for glucose. Thus, there is a three-part sequence of fuel utilization in prolonged exercise. First, the muscle burns its own storage of glucose; then it takes glucose that has been released from storage in the liver; finally the main fuel source becomes free fatty acids, which are released into the bloodstream from the body's fat stores.

After exercise ceases, blood flow to the muscle decreases, but the uptake of glucose remains three to four times the resting level for nearly an hour. This attempt to replenish muscle glucose applies to the liver, but for even longer periods of time. Insulin levels rise after exercise to facilitate this response. However, *during exercise, insulin levels decrease, yet muscle uptake of glucose is enhanced!* This indicates that the muscle uptake of glucose during exercise does not require increased insulin. The exact mechanism by which exercising muscle can take glucose from the bloodstream and use it is not fully understood. However, it is this very occurrence that is largely responsible for the reduced insulin requirements and improved glucose tolerance that come with exercise.

Exercise does pose a potential problem for the insulin-dependent diabetic. The release of insulin from a subcutaneous injection is steady and does not fall off during exercise as it does in the nondiabetic. In fact, if the insulin is injected in an exercised site, such as the leg in a runner, insulin release is markedly enhanced by exercise. This means that the liver will not release glucose into the bloodstream, whereas in the normal person, decline in insulin levels during exercise triggers the liver to release glucose into the bloodstream. Thus, the release of stored glycogen in the diabetic's liver as glucose in the bloodstream is reduced. This is partially offset by the fact that the diabetic's ability to manufacture glucose is enhanced. However, the net effect is reduced liver glucose output, thus rendering the insulin-dependent diabetic potentially at risk for hypoglycemia or low blood sugar unless he either decreases his intake of insulin or increases his intake of carbohydrates before engaging in unusually strenuous prolonged exercise. Most diabetics would find either alternative quite desirable.

Exercise, therefore, affords a reduction in insulin re-

quirements and liberalization of carbohydrate intake in the insulin-dependent diabetic. For many adult-onset diabetics, exercise can eliminate insulin requirements entirely and return glucose tolerance to normal. In a word, it "cures" the disease.

It is no surprise that all of the diabetic marathoners who have been interviewed indicated that vigorous exercise, in their case daily running, markedly enhanced diabetic control. Exercise reduced their daily insulin requirements from 10 percent to 50 percent. All expressed the need for additional insulin during periods of enforced inactivity. Marathoner Guy Hornsby stated, "My insulin requirements are directly related to my weekly mileage. With no running, my diet of twenty-two hundred calories must be supplemented with sixty units of U-100 Lente insulin. At my current level of running, approximately fifty miles per week, I have to take only thirty-five units. My lowest intake has been twenty-five units and this was achieved with an excess of eighty miles per week." Another marathoner, Jim Kirk, noted, "In the summer months, when I am training harder, I require only one injection in the morning. On the other hand, during the winter, I require two injections daily." These comments are typical, and they remind me of a backpacking experience with teenage insulin-dependent diabetics, during which most were able to cut their daily insulin dose by 75 percent. These hikers, who were involved with day-long exercise, ate small snacks every hour to guard against hypoglycemia, as do skiers, canoers, and other sports participants.

Well-regulated diabetics have an exercise energy metabolism that is not different in principle from that of similarly trained nondiabetics. Exercise reduces the level of blood sugar by enhancing muscle glucose uptake muscle in diabetics and nondiabetics alike. The insulin receptors in diabetics have been shown to become more sensitive in response to exercise. Thus, even when the level of circulating insulin is extremely low, glucose utilization by muscle and other tissues is increased. This is true in both juvenile- and adult-onset diabetics. Exercise also enhances the utilization of free fatty acids (FFA), *ketone bodies,* as well as glycogen in liver and working muscle.

Furthermore, moderate to intense exercise increases tolerance for glucose in both the nondiabetic and the diabetic. This is believed to be a result of the not yet fully understood effects that exercise has on glucose metabolism for as long as twenty-four to forty-eight hours after the period of exertion. During this postexercise period, the replenishment of muscle and liver glycogen occurs. As compared to the preexercise or resting state, a greater proportion of the sugar and starch (carbohydrate) the diabetic eats goes toward replenishing muscle glycogen. Since glucose uptake by muscle and glycogen resynthesis in the muscle and the liver requires a minimal concentration of insulin, the diabetic experiences an improvement in glucose tolerance while insulin requirements are diminished.

A side benefit of sustained vigorous activity can be a less strict diet. Marathoner Gerald Janusz is one diabetic who found this to be true: "After I started running, I needed more calories. It became clear that I could be somewhat more free with my diet because of the exercise. Gradually, I put the exchange system aside and became less concerned about calorie counting. I had always eaten well-balanced meals and continue to do so daily. One of the advantages of a regular running program is that I am able to eat normal meals." While your diabetes may not be this stable even with daily exercise, a tendency toward stability is to be anticipated. Said another diabetic marathoner, Mark Collins, "The running, perhaps, has given me more liberties with diet than nonexercising diabetics have."

Insulin is necessary for transporting the building blocks of protein (amino acids) into the muscle. In prolonged starvation and uncontrolled diabetes, the muscle protein, when broken down during exercise, is not replenished, which causes the muscle to begin wasting away. When the disease is controlled, however, increased exercise brings on rapid muscle growth (hypertrophy). Thus, diabetics can engage in every sport, includ-

31

ing weight lifting and body building where increasing muscle bulk is of paramount importance.

The message for the diabetic is loud and clear. *Exercise is mandatory for maximal control of your disease, and daily exercise will very likely retard the development of vascular complications. Your cardiovascular system can become conditioned as quickly as that of the nondiabetic. There is no exercise you should avoid. Your only risk is in developing hypoglycemia with sustained exercise over forty minutes of uninterrupted activity, and your carbohydrate intake and/or insulin administration can be adjusted accordingly.* There are diabetics running in marathons and actively pursuing every competitive endurance sport.

4.

Your Doctor and Your Level of Fitness

HOW TO CHOOSE YOUR DOCTOR

Most diabetics are under medical supervision, but is your doctor the one to prescribe your exercise program? It goes without saying that the physician must not only be qualified in diabetes management but also be knowledgeable about aerobic exercise (exertion at a level below one's maximum ability to consume oxygen). Ask yourself and your doctor these simple questions. A high proportion of yes answers may indicate that a second opinion is advisable.

QUESTIONS FOR YOU AND YOUR DOCTOR

1. Did your doctor ask you to curtail your physical activities when your diabetes was diagnosed?
2. Did your doctor place any physical restrictions on your life?
3. Does your doctor proscribe aerobic exercise programs?
4. Does your doctor never discuss the "wellness" concept and preventive medicine?

5. Have you and your doctor never discussed the treatment triad of diet, exercise, and insulin and how they interact?
6. Is your doctor physically passive himself?
7. Is your doctor obese?
8. Does your doctor smoke cigarettes?
9. Does your doctor paint a bleak outlook for normal life?
10. Does your doctor prescribe rigid insulin requirements and place none of the diabetes management on you?
11. Does your doctor seem distant and difficult to communicate with on a personal basis?
12. Is your doctor not a member of the American College of Sports Medicine?
13. Does your doctor never read any of the sports medicine journals?

If the answer to one or more of the questions is yes, you possibly have the wrong doctor for your diabetes management and exercise program.

Having the "right" doctor is important for maximal diabetes management, but it is even more crucial to your outlook on life and your best emotional health. Of the diabetic marathoners interviewed, surprisingly, most indicated that they regarded diabetes as having little emotional impact on their lives. Without exception, the majority who felt this way all received extensive information and education about diabetes from their physician. In many cases, this included an initial period of hospitalization, during which insulin administration was learned, initial requirements determined for diet, exercise, and insulin, and a myriad of questions answered. The belief that diabetes has little effect on diabetics emotionally is well expressed by runner Jim Kirk: "As far as an emotional impact upon being told I was diabetic, I do not think I felt any. The nurses and doctors around me made every effort to explain the disease and how to live with it. They provided me with all kinds of literature on diabetes, and it was quite a learning experience for me."

Marathoner Gerald Janusz said: "After spending six days in the hospital and receiving a brief but comprehensive education about the care of the diabetic, I felt no particular apprehension about my disease. I was quite sure that my life would not be drastically changed and I would be able to take care of myself."

Runner Guy Hornsby told us: "Dr. Luce explained my condition to me and was very supportive of my participation in sports. He told me I could try any sport I wanted to as long as I stuck to my diet and medication. He followed me closely throughout high school and made adjustments to my treatment but did not prevent me from playing any specific sport."

However, it is also true that those few who described the onset of diabetes as being emotionally traumatic *all* described a lack of information regarding diabetes from their physician. Bill Royston spoke for this minority when he said: "The onset of diabetes was at the age of twenty-five. This was quite a traumatic blow since I had never so much as been in the hospital and had always taken my good health for granted. The bad news was compounded by my lack of knowledge of the condition and a country doctor who gave me little idea of what to expect."

How do you find the right doctor? There are no absolute answers. In general, you will do better with a specialist in diabetes who is himself in good physical condition, a sports enthusiast knowledgeable in aerobic exercise, and, perhaps above all else, one with whom you can establish a meaningful, comfortable rapport. Do not be apologetic or afraid to seek a second opinion: Your life is at stake! Realize that no worthwhile, mature physician will ever be offended by a patient seeking a second opinion. This is equally true for all specialists. It is a fact that doctors themselves strongly prefer to have patients with whom they have little rapport cared for by other physicians. Often the doctors are timid in admitting this, feeling some inadequacy on their part, but they are greatly relieved when the patient takes the initiative and seeks another opinion.

DETERMINING YOUR LEVEL OF FITNESS

Before the diabetic begins an exercise program, he or she should undergo a thorough physical examination. It should include a family history of relevant medical problems and familial traits, a blood lipid profile, resting blood pressure, and a resting 12-lead electrocardiogram (EKG). If you are over thirty-five, an exercise 12-lead EKG is also recommended. It is only by stressing the heart in this manner that irregular heartbeats and signs of heart strain can be detected. If heart irregularities appear, your exercise program may have to be greatly modified to avoid the risk of heart attack. Gradually, as your stress EKG improves, your level of physical conditioning can be advanced.

The stress electrocardiogram is especially important for the diabetic who has previously been sedentary and had little regular exercise, who has a family history of heart attack, or who has been taking insulin more than ten years. The test is least necessary in the diabetic who already engages in daily aerobic exercise for more than thirty minutes, but it is still recommended for such an individual over thirty-five who has been insulin-dependent more than ten years.

Your maximal heart rate, that rate of exertion that leaves you totally out of breath, and associated blood pressure should also be recorded.

Finally, it is helpful, although not essential, to have your maximum oxygen uptake recorded. Many community hospitals and virtually all large teaching medical centers carry out this test. It permits an objective comparison of your present level of fitness with age-related tables, giving an accurate indication of not only your present fitness but your performance capability. By repeating the examination at specific intervals after beginning an exercise program, your rate of fitness improvement can be documented. Obviously, such a test is immensely useful to coaches and competitive athletes planning training programs.

Although a test of maximal oxygen consumption (VO_2 max.) is the most precise measurement of one's fitness, several practical considerations make this test undesirable for all but the superbly conditioned athlete. First, since the endpoint is exhaustion, one must consider whether the subject quit short of exhaustion because of low tolerance to physical discomfort, lack of motivation, or even fear of a coronary.

Because of these drawbacks, *submaximal oxygen consumption testing* is the test most used to determine fitness. It is based on the fact that oxygen consumption and heart rate both increase in a straight line in response to increased physical effort. Thus, this test involves physical effort, usually either running on a treadmill or riding a bicycle ergometer, that brings the heart rate up approximately to 50 percent and 75 percent of one's age-computed maximal level as read from tables. Your oxygen consumption is measured at these two levels and from them your maximal VO_2 max. is calculated. There is also a simplification of the submaximal test that uses tables to relate heart rate and oxygen consumption. Here, heart rate is plotted against work load to obtain a predicted VO_2 max. from a table of average equivalents. This is accurate within a range of 10 percent. This test eliminates the need to collect and analyze expired air and, thus, becomes practical in an office setting.

Ideally, your complete fitness exam should include an assessment of body composition, lean body mass versus body fat. The only precise method of determining body fat is the immersion technique, but this is unavailable except in certain exercise laboratories. However, an adequate alternative technique you can perform on yourself involves measuring your body fat at

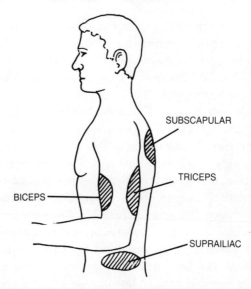

SUBSCAPULAR

TRICEPS

BICEPS

SUPRAILIAC

Figure 2. The Four Body Fat Sites

four sites: behind the triceps muscle (back of the upper arm), over the biceps muscle, at the inferior angle of the scapula, and the suprailiac (vertical skin fold on the crest of the hip. (See Figure 2.) Use a caliper to measure the skin fold thickness in each area in millimeters, and then add up the total millimeters: This is your fat index. Table 3 allows you to compute your percent body fat (plus or minus 5 percent) and gives suggested percents at various ages. Repeat these measurements as your fitness schedule progresses. You can anticipate a 20 percent to 25 percent reduction in skin-fold fat measurements, even if you have not lost any total body weight. If dieting is used in conjunction with exercise, a much greater reduction of body fat will occur.

Since muscle weighs more than fat, it is possible to sustain a given weight during an exercise program and still lose considerable body fat. This is especially true for the already lean person. Those underweight may even experience a slight weight

TABLE 3
FAT CONTENT, AS PERCENTAGE OF BODY WEIGHT, FOR THE SUM OF FOUR SKIN FOLDS

SKIN FOLDS, MM	MALES (AGE IN YEARS)				FEMALES (AGE IN YEARS)			
	17–29	30–39	40–49	50+	16–29	30–39	40–49	50+
15	4.8	—	—	—	10.5	—	—	—
20	8.1	12.2	12.2	12.6	14.1	17.0	19.8	21.4
25	10.5	14.2	15.0	15.6	16.8	19.4	22.2	24.0
30	12.9	16.2	17.7	18.6	19.5	21.8	24.5	26.6
35	14.7	17.7	19.6	20.8	21.5	23.7	26.4	28.5
40	16.4	19.2	21.4	22.0	28.4	25.5	28.2	30.3
45	17.7	20.4	23.0	24.7	25.0	26.9	29.6	31.9
50	19.0	21.5	24.6	26.5	26.5	28.2	31.0	33.4
55	20.1	22.5	25.9	27.9	27.8	29.4	32.1	34.6
60	21.2	23.5	27.1	29.2	29.1	30.6	33.2	35.7
65	22.2	24.3	28.2	30.4	30.2	31.6	34.1	36.7
70	23.1	25.1	29.3	31.6	31.2	32.5	35.0	37.7
75	24.0	25.9	30.3	32.7	32.2	33.4	35.9	38.7
80	24.8	26.6	31.2	33.8	35.1	34.3	36.7	39.6
85	25.8	27.2	32.1	34.8	34.0	35.1	37.5	40.4
90	26.2	27.8	33.0	35.8	34.8	35.8	38.3	41.2
95	26.9	28.4	33.7	36.6	35.6	36.5	39.0	41.9
100	27.6	29.0	34.4	37.4	36.4	37.2	39.7	42.6
105	28.2	29.6	35.1	38.2	37.1	37.9	40.4	43.3
110	28.8	30.1	35.8	39.0	37.8	38.6	41.0	43.9
115	29.4	30.6	36.4	39.7	38.4	39.1	41.5	44.5
120	30.0	31.1	37.0	40.4	39.0	39.6	42.0	45.1
125	30.5	31.5	37.6	41.1	39.6	40.1	42.5	45.7
130	31.0	31.9	38.2	41.8	40.2	40.6	43.0	46.2
135	31.5	32.3	38.7	42.4	40.8	41.1	43.5	46.7
140	32.0	32.7	39.2	43.0	41.3	41.6	44.0	47.2
145	32.5	33.1	39.7	43.6	41.8	42.1	44.5	47.7
150	32.9	33.5	40.2	44.1	42.3	42.6	45.0	48.2
155	33.3	33.9	40.7	44.6	42.8	43.1	45.4	48.7
160	33.7	34.3	41.2	45.1	43.3	43.6	45.8	49.2
165	34.1	34.6	41.6	45.6	43.7	44.0	46.2	49.6
170	34.5	34.8	42.0	46.1	44.1	44.4	46.6	50.0
MAXIMUM DESIRABLE PERCENTAGE	12.0	20.0	22.0	25.0	23.0	27.0	30.0	34.0

gain as muscle is added. This principle applies to the conditioning of the cardiovascular-pulmonary system.

Finally, to increase the efficiency of the heart and lungs, it is essential to perform continuous rhythmic exercises long enough to stress the cardiovascular-pulmonary system. Thus, brisk walking, jogging, bicycling, cross-country skiing should be maintained until the body begins to perspire and the pulse rate rises above 130 beats per minute for several minutes. Within ten minutes after exertion, your pulse rate should return to normal and you should not feel fatigued. If the return to normal does not occur, you are advancing too fast.

5.

Your Graded Exercise Program

FINDING YOUR FITNESS LEVEL

Although I urge you to see a qualified physician to receive a fitness examination and a subsequent exercise prescription, I know not all of you will or can comply. Before you proceed with the tests and programs described in the rest of this chapter, let me reiterate my recommendation that you first obtain a fitness examination and commence the program under a qualified physician's supervision.

You can determine your own level of fitness by simple easy tests. The walk test is the easiest. The intent of the walk test is to determine how many minutes, up to a total of ten, you can walk briskly on a flat surface without experiencing undue shortness of breath or discomfort. If you can walk briskly for only three minutes or less, you are at level 3, the Basic Level. If you can easily exceed three minutes, but cannot comfortably walk ten minutes, you are at Level 2, or Moderate Fitness. If you can easily walk ten minutes, then you may be at Level 1. To determine if you are at Level 1, an additional test can be attempted; it consists of walking and jogging. Alternately walk 50 steps and jog 50 steps for a total of six minutes. Walk at a rate of at least 120 steps per minute and jog at a rate of 144 steps per minute. If you must stop this test before six minutes have elapsed, you are a Level 2. If you can easily complete the six-minute test, you are at Level 1. If you can complete twelve minutes of this test, you can move beyond Level 1 to any of the endurance sports (jogging, swimming, cycling, and cross-country skiing) listed in Table 6.

To be of maximal value for diabetes control, your exercises should be done daily. A half hour should be sufficient time. Start easily and slowly and increase the tempo and number of repetitions. If you feel a little stiff, do not let this deter you. However, if you experience actual pain that does not disappear within forty-eight hours, don't use that exercise until medical clearance is given and the exercise can be resumed without pain. The exercises for each level—1, 2, and 3— should be carried out in the sequence given because both a warm-up and cooling-off period are built into each series. The cooling-off period has recently received much attention in the Olympic games. It has been shown that the cooling-off phase allows muscles to be drained of lactic acids, the products of aerobic metabolism, and it is the best way to prepare the body for the next day's strenuous activity. If possible, keep a log or record of the exercises you perform, how many repetitions you do, and how much time you require. Many find that doing the exercises to music makes them more enjoyable. Others find that watching the evening TV news or listening to the radio while exercising relieves boredom. The exercises can be done alone or with family and friends. Clothing should be loose, comfortable, and quite stretchable rather than restrictive. Shoes should have no heels and nonskid soles. The only reason you should not exercise on a given day is if your diabetes is in poor control and there are 4+ sugar and ketones in your urine. As discussed in chapter 4, diabetic ketosis will likely be augmented by vigorous exercise. In this instance, it is best to adjust diet and insulin to bring your diabetes under control before exercising, even if it means skipping a day here and there.

YOUR OWN EXERCISE PROGRAM BASED ON YOUR LEVEL OF FITNESS

LEVEL 3: THE BASIC LEVEL

You should attempt to complete the entire sequence of exercises in level 3 without rest periods of more than two minutes. If necessary, however, as you begin, take a longer rest period, but try to finish the entire sequence. An indication of improvement in your level of fitness will be your ability to complete the sequence comfortably in less time. Never execute an exercise in a jerky manner to increase speed. All exercises should be done as smoothly and comfortably as possible.

1. Walk; 3 minutes (Exercise 1)
2. Bend and Stretch; 2 increasing to 10 repetitions (Exercise 3)
3. Rotate Head; 2 increasing to 10 repetitions each way (Exercise 4)
4. Body Bender; 2 increasing to 5 repetitions (Exercise 5)
5. Back Flattener; 2 increasing to 5 repetitions (Exercise 6)
6. Wall Press; 2 increasing to 5 repetitions (Exercise 7)
7. Arm Circles; 5 repetitions each way (Exercise 9)
8. Wing Stretcher; 2 increasing to 5 repetitions (Exercise 11)
9. Single Knee Raise; 3 increasing to 10 repetitions (Exercise 13)
10. Straight Arm and Leg Stretch; 2 increasing to 5 repetitions (Exercise 18)
11. Heel-Toe Walk (Exercise 19)
12. Side Leg Raise; 2 increasing to 5 repetitions each leg (Exercise 23)

13. Partial Sit-up; 2 increasing to 10 repetitions (Exercise 24)
14. Alternate Walk-Jog; 1 to 3 minutes (Exercise 30)
15. Walk; 1 to 3 minutes (Exercise 1)

For the first week do the fewest repetitions or shortest duration of time shown for each exercise. If after a week you still find that this level requires a strenuous effort, do not increase the duration or repetitions. Only when you feel comfortable with an exercise where a range of repetitions is given should you slowly increase the number by one additional repetition per week. When you can carry out the maximum number of repetitions indicated for each exercise without resting between, you are ready to move on to Level 2.

LEVEL 2: MODERATE FITNESS

For the Level 2 exercise program, you should proceed in a manner similar to Level 3. Start at the fewest number of repetitions and gradually advance a repetition at a time until you are capable of performing the highest continuous number of repetitions of each exercise. When this can be accomplished without straining or undue fatigue, you are ready to advance to Level 1.

1. Walk; 3 minutes (Exercise 1)
2. Bend and Stretch; 10 repetitions (Exercise 3)
3. Rotate Head; 10 repetitions each way (Exercise 4)
4. Body Bender; 5 increasing to 10 repetitions (Exercise 5)
5. Back Flattener; 5 increasing to 10 repetitions (Exercise 6)
6. Wall Press; 5 repetitions (Exercise 7)
7. Arm Circles; 5 increasing to 10 repetitions (Exercise 9)

8. Half Knee Bend; 5 increasing to 10 repetitions (Exercise 10)
9. Wing Stretcher; 5 increasing to 10 repetitions (Exercise 11)
10. Single Knee Hug; 3 increasing to 10 repetitions (Exercise 14)
11. Single Leg Raise; 3 increasing to 10 repetitions (Exercise 16)
12. Straight Arm and Leg Stretch; 5 repetitions (Exercise 18)
13. Heel-Toe Beam Walk (Exercise 20)
14. Knee Push-up; 2 increasing to 10 repetitions (Exercise 22)
15. Side Leg Raise; 2 increasing to 10 repetitions each leg (Exercise 23)
16. Advanced Sit-up; 2 increasing to 10 repetitions each leg (Exercise 25)
17. Sitting Bend; 2 increasing to 5 repetitions (Exercise 27)
18. Deep Knee Bend; 2 increasing to 5 repetitions (Exercise 29)
19. Alternate Walk-Jog; 3 to 6 minutes (Exercise 30)
20. Walk; 1 to 3 minutes (Exercise 1)

LEVEL 1: GOOD FITNESS

The same directions, starting with the fewest repetitions and gradually increasing, apply for Level 1. When you can perform the maximum repetitions without rest periods, you can either continue to increase the number of repetitions and speed of their execution or advance to other more vigorous exercises and sports as discussed in chapter 8.

1. Alternate Walk-Jog; 3 minutes (Exercise 2)
2. Bend and Stretch; 10 repetitions (Exercise 3)

3. Rotate Head; 10 repetitions each way (Exercise 4)
4. Body Bender; 10 repetitions (Exercise 5)
5. Back Flattener with legs extended; 10 repetitions (Exercise 6)
6. Wall Press; 5 repetitions (Exercise 7)
7. Posture Check; 5 repetitions (Exercise 8)
8. Arm Circles; 10 increasing to 15 repetitions each way (Exercise 9)
9. Half Knee Bend; 10 increasing to 20 repetitions (Exercise 10)
10. Wing Stretcher; 10 increasing to 20 repetitions (Exercise 11)
11. Wall Push-up; 10 repetitions (Exercise 12)
12. Double Knee Hug; 3 increasing to 10 repetitions (Exercise 15)
13. Single Leg Raise and Knee Hug; 3 increasing to 10 repetitions (Exercise 17)
14. Straight Arm and Leg Stretch; 5 repetitions (Exercise 18)
15. Heel-Toe Beam Walk (Exercise 20)
16. Hop; 5 repetitions on each foot (Exercise 21)
17. Knee Push-up; 3 increasing to 10 repetitions (Exercise 22)
18. Side Leg Raise; 10 repetitions each leg (Exercise 23)
19. Advanced Modified Sit-up; 2 increasing to 10 repetitions (Exercise 26)
20. Sitting Bend; 5 increasing to 10 repetitions (Exercise 27)
21. Diver's Stance; hold 10 seconds (Exercise 28)
22. Deep Knee Bend; 5 increasing to 10 repetitions (Exercise 29)
23. Alternate Walk-Jog; 5 minutes (Exercise 30)
24. Walk; 3 minutes (Exercise 1)

EXERCISES USED IN ALL THREE BASIC LEVELS

EXERCISE 1. WALK

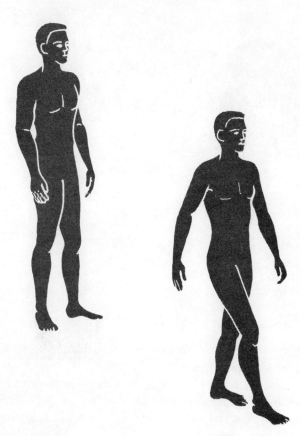

OBJECTIVE: An excellent warm-up exercise to loosen muscles and prepare you for the ensuing exercises.

BASIC EXERCISE: Stand erect and be well balanced on the balls of your feet. Begin walking rapidly on a level surface.

EXERCISE 2. ALTERNATE WALK-JOG

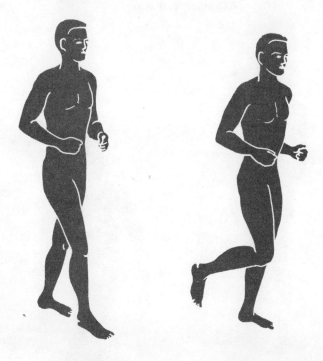

OBJECTIVE: Warm-up exercise for more advanced exercises; good for legs and circulation.

BASIC EXERCISE: Stand erect, as for walking, with arms held flexed and forearms roughly parallel to the floor. Begin walking for 50 steps, then break into a slow run (jog) for 50 steps. When jogging, stride easily, landing on your heels and rolling to push off on your toes. This heel-toe movement is in contrast to a fast run where you land and stay on the balls of your feet. Arms should swing freely from the shoulders in opposition to the legs. Breathing should be deep but never labored to the point of gasping. Continue for 3 minutes.

EXERCISE 3. BEND AND STRETCH

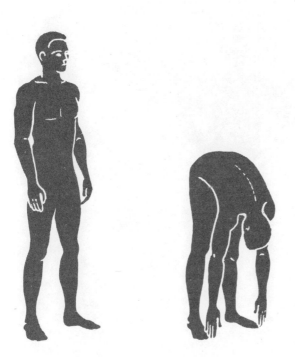

OBJECTIVE: To loosen and stretch primarily the back, hamstring, and calf muscles.

BASIC EXERCISE: Stand erect, with your feet shoulder-width apart. Slowly bend forward at the waist and touch the fingers of your outstretched arms to your toes, bending your knees to whatever degree is necessary to accomplish this maneuver. The maximal effort is achieved when the knees can remain locked. Return slowly and smoothly to the starting position.

EXERCISE 4. ROTATE HEAD

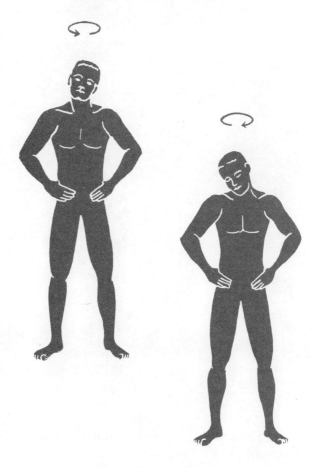

OBJECTIVE: To loosen and relax the muscles of the neck and to firm up the throat and chin line.

BASIC EXERCISE: Stand erect, with your feet shoulder-width apart and your hands on your hips. Slowly, in a smooth motion, rotate your head in a full circle, stretching from left to right; then slowly rotate your head in a full circle stretching from right to left.

EXERCISE 5. BODY BENDER

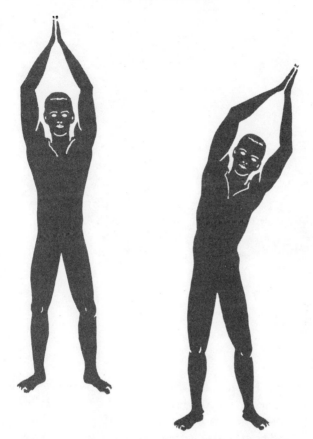

OBJECTIVE: To stretch arm, trunk, and leg muscles.

BASIC EXERCISE: Stand erect, with your feet shoulder-width apart and your hands extended overhead with your finger-tips touching as in a praying hand posture. Bend at the waist, stretching gently and slowly sideward to the left as far as possible while keeping your hands together and your arms extended straight; return to starting position; repeat same movements to the right.

51

EXERCISE 6. BACK FLATTENER

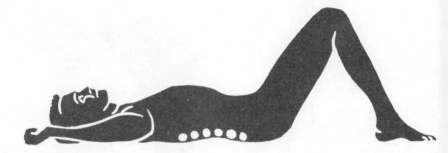

OBJECTIVE: Strengthen gluteal (buttock) and abdominal muscles and flatten the lower back, help lumbar lordosis. BASIC EXERCISE: Lie on your back on padded floor with knees well bent. Relax with arms above your head. A small pillow may be placed under your head if desired. Now squeeze your buttocks together as if trying to hold a piece of paper between them. At the same time suck in and tighten the muscles of your abdomen. You should feel your back flatten against the floor. This is the *flat back position*. Hold this position for a count of ten (10 seconds); relax and then repeat the exercise three times in the beginning. Gradually attempt to increase to 20 repetitions.

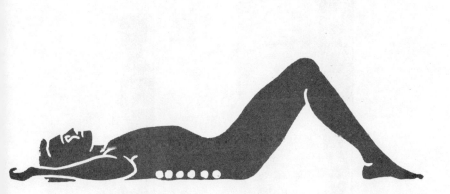

ADVANCED MODIFICATIONS

BUTTOCK RAISE: After the basic exercise has been done for a week or more, additional flattening can be achieved by doing the exercise with the buttocks slightly raised off the floor (1 to 2 inches) at the time the buttocks are squeezed and the abdomen tensed. Hold for the count of ten; relax and repeat.

LEGS EXTENDED: After several weeks of the basic exercise, gradually do the exercise with the knees less and less bent, until you can execute the exercise with your legs straight. The buttock raise need not be combined with this modification.

EXERCISE 7. WALL PRESS

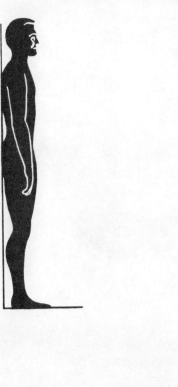

OBJECTIVE: To promote good body alignment and posture while strengthening abdominal muscles.

BASIC EXERCISE: Stand erect, with your head and neck in a neutral position, your back against the wall, and your heels three inches away from the wall. Suck in your stomach and press your lower back flat against the wall. Hold this position for six seconds; relax and return to the starting position. Your lower back should continuously be in contact with the wall and your head and neck should not extend backward.

EXERCISE 8. POSTURE CHECK

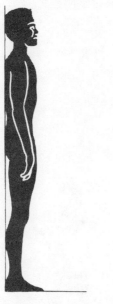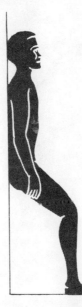

OBJECTIVE: To help you stand and walk correctly. To help you in determining if your exercise program is accomplishing its goals.

BASIC EXERCISE: Stand with your back to the wall, pressing your heels, buttocks, shoulders, and head against the wall. You should not be able to feel any space between your lower back and the wall; if you can, your back is too arched and not flat. Move your feet forward, bending your knees so that your back slides a few inches down the wall. Now, again, squeeze your buttocks and tighten your abdominal muscles flattening your lower back against the wall. While holding this position, walk your feet back so you slide up the wall. Now, standing straight, walk away from the wall and around the room. Return to the wall and back up to it to be certain you've kept the proper posture.

55

EXERCISE 9. ARM CIRCLES

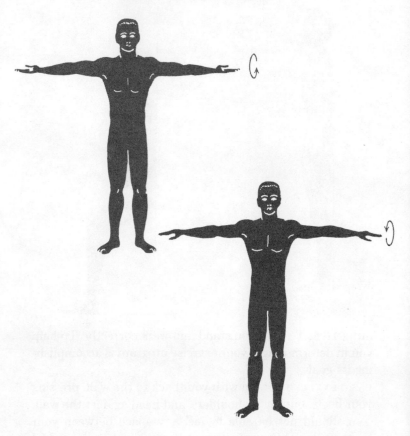

OBJECTIVE: To strengthen the muscles of the shoulder while keeping the joint flexible.

BASIC EXERCISE: Stand erect, with your arms outstretched sideward at shoulder height, palms up. While keeping your head erect, make small circular movements with your hands backward as if inscribing a perfect circle, then reverse and, now with your palms down, carry out the circular movements in a forward circle.

EXERCISE 10. HALF KNEE BEND

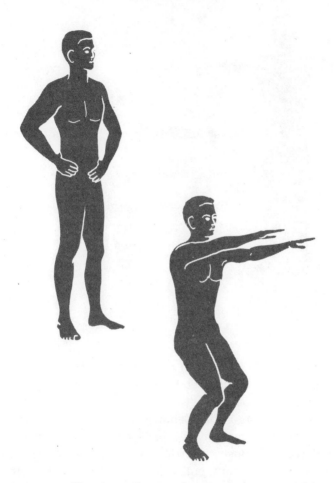

OBJECTIVE: To strengthen and stretch your quadriceps (upper front thigh) muscles while improving your balance.
BASIC EXERCISE: Stand erect, with your hands on your hips. While extending your arms forward, palms down, bend your knees halfway. Keep your heels on the floor, pause, and return to the starting position.

EXERCISE 11. WING STRETCHER

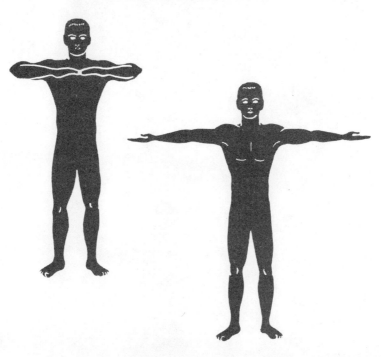

OBJECTIVE: To strengthen the muscles of the upper back and shoulders while stretching the chest muscles and promoting good posture.

BASIC EXERCISE: While standing erect, bend your arms in front of your chest, with your elbows at shoulder height and your extended fingertips touching. Count one, two, three; on each count, pull your elbows backward as far as possible while keeping your arms at shoulder height and then returning to the starting position. Then swing your arms (on count four) outward and sideward, shoulder height, palms up, and return to the starting position. As you do this exercise, count to yourself one and two and three and four, etc.

EXERCISE 12. WALL PUSH-UP

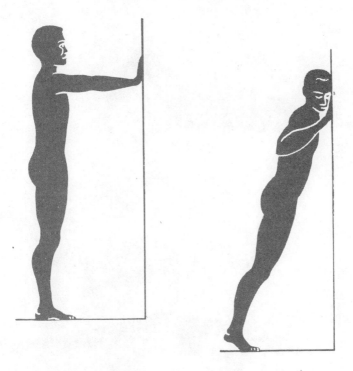

OBJECTIVE: To strengthen arm, shoulder, and upper back muscles while stretching the chest and posterior thigh muscles.

BASIC EXERCISE: Stand erect, squarely facing the wall, with your feet about six inches apart and your arms extended straight in front, with your palms on the wall lightly bearing weight. Slowly bend your elbows and lower your body toward the wall, turning your head to the side until your cheek almost touches the wall. Then slowly push away from the wall, extending your elbows while returning to the initial position. Then slowly repeat, this time turning your head to the opposite side.

EXERCISE 13. SINGLE KNEE RAISE

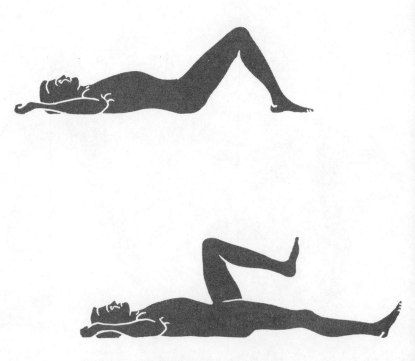

OBJECTIVE: To stretch lower back, hip flexor, and hamstring (posterior thigh) muscles.

BASIC EXERCISE: Lie on your back on a padded floor, with your arms above your head and your knees bent. Tighten your buttocks and abdominal muscles as in Exercise 6. Then raise one knee over your chest toward your chin as far as possible, hold for ten seconds, then return to starting position and relax a few seconds before repeating with the opposite leg. Start with three repetitions of each knee gradually advancing to ten.

EXERCISE 14. SINGLE KNEE HUG

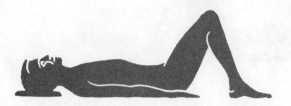

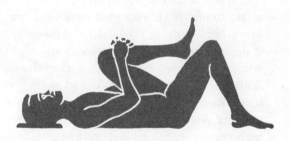

OBJECTIVE: Same as single knee raise.

BASIC EXERCISE: The single knee hug is essentially the same exercise as the single knee raise, except that the hands are not placed above the head but rather around the knee to be raised. The arms are used to pull (raise) the knee higher over the chest than was possible in Exercise 13. This produces greater stretching of the lower back and hamstrings.

EXERCISE 15. DOUBLE KNEE HUG

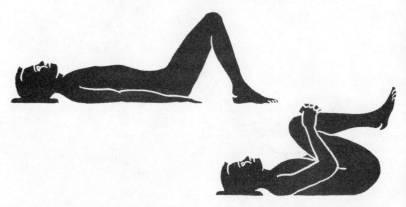

OBJECTIVE: To stretch lower back and hamstring muscles and strengthen abdominal and hip-flexing muscles.

BASIC EXERCISE: Lie on your back on a covered floor with knees bent, arms at your side, and pillow under your head, if desired. Tighten your buttocks and abdominal muscles so that your lower back is flat against the floor. Now grasp both knees with your hands and raise them slowly over your chest as far as possible. Hold ten seconds, return to starting position, relax a few seconds, then repeat. Start with three repetitions and gradually build to ten.

ADVANCED MODIFICATION: After a month or more of the basic exercise, attempt the double knee hug starting with both legs extended straight. Tense your buttocks and abdomen, and then, taking care to keep the back flat, bend both knees, grasp knees with hands and raise over your chest, hold ten seconds and return to starting position to relax before repeating. The lower back tends to arch when the knee is lifted and lowered. If you cannot do this with your back against the floor, you are not yet ready for this modification and should resume the basic knees bent position. This extended-leg starting position strengthens both the hip-flexing and abdominal muscles.

EXERCISE 16. SINGLE LEG RAISE

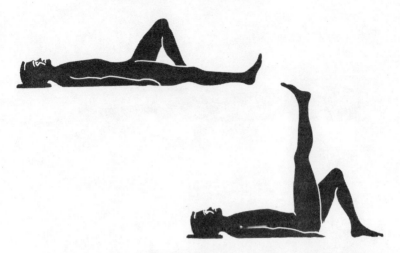

OBJECTIVE: To stretch lower back and hamstring muscles and strengthen abdominal and hip-flexing muscles.

BASIC EXERCISE: Lie on your back on a covered floor with one knee bent and one leg straight, arms at your side, and a pillow under your head, if desired. Tighten your buttocks and abdominal muscles, then slowly raise the straight leg, keeping the leg straight and your back flat. Raise the leg as far as comfortably possible, then slowly lower the leg, keeping it straight and your back flat to the floor. Relax a few seconds, and then repeat with the other leg. Start with three repetitions of each leg and gradually increase to ten.

ADVANCED MODIFICATION: After a month or more, attempt the single leg raise starting with both legs extended straight. Tense your buttocks and lower back, and with your back flat and legs out straight, raise one leg up as far as possible. As the leg is raised, your back may not remain flat. Check by using your hand to see if your back lifts from the floor when the leg is lifted and lowered. If it does, resume the basic exercise with one knee bent.

EXERCISE 17. SINGLE LEG RAISE AND KNEE HUG

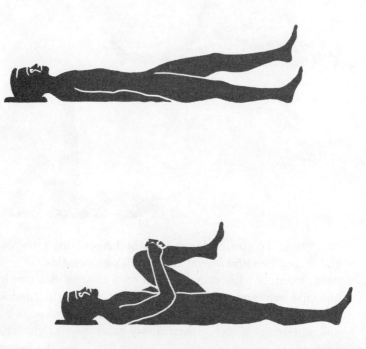

OBJECTIVE: To strengthen lower back and abdominal muscles while increasing flexibility of hip and knee joints.

BASIC EXERCISE: Raise extended left leg about twelve inches off the floor; slowly bend your knee and move it toward your chest as far as possible using your abdominal, hip, and leg muscles. Then place both hands around your knee and pull it slowly toward your chest as far as possible. Slowly extend your leg to the position twelve inches off the floor, then return to the starting position. Repeat 3 to 5 times with each leg. Do the number desired with the left leg, then switch and repeat with the right leg.

EXERCISE 18. STRAIGHT ARM AND LEG STRETCH

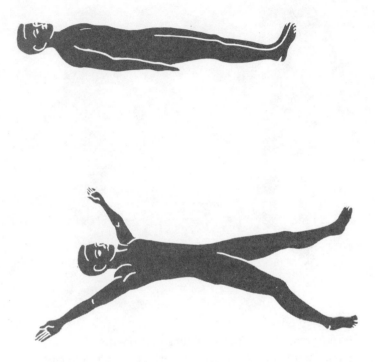

OBJECTIVE: To strengthen abdominal muscles while stretching the muscles of the arms.

BASIC EXERCISE: Lie on your back, legs extended, feet together, arms at your side, your buttocks and abdomen tensed so that your back is flat against the floor. Slowly move arms and legs outward along the floor as far as possible, hold a moment, and slowly return to the starting position. Repetitions as indicated for each level.

EXERCISE 19. HEEL-TOE WALK

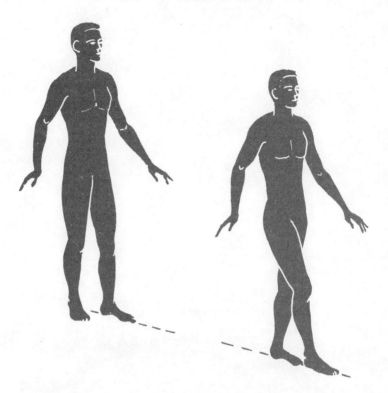

OBJECTIVE: To improve balance and posture.

BASIC EXERCISE: Stand erect, with abdomen and buttocks tensed and your left foot along a straight line and your hands held out from your body to aid in balance. Walk ten steps along the straight line by placing the right foot directly in front of the left, with the right heel touching the left great toe. Then alternate feet, placing the left in front of the right, heel-to-toe. When ten such steps in a straight line have been taken, stop; then return to the starting position by walking backward along the same line, alternately placing one foot behind the other, toe-to-heel.

EXERCISE 20. HEEL-TOE BEAM WALK

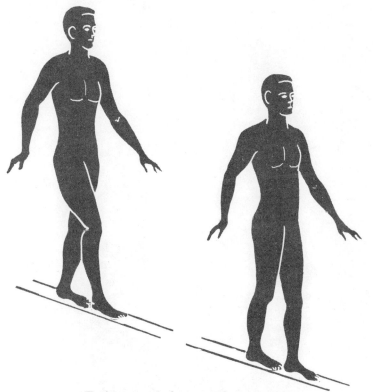

OBJECTIVE: To improve balance and posture.

BASIC EXERCISE: Level 2 will walk ten steps on a 2-inch-high by 6-inch-wide board placed flat on the floor. Level 1 on a 2-inch-high by 4-inch-wide board placed flat on the floor. Walk ten steps along the board by placing the right foot directly in front of the left with the right heel touching the left great toe. Then alternate feet, placing the left foot in front of the right, heel-to-toe. When ten such steps have been taken, stop, then return to the starting position by walking backward along the same board, alternately placing one foot behind the other, toe-to-heel.

EXERCISE 21. HOP

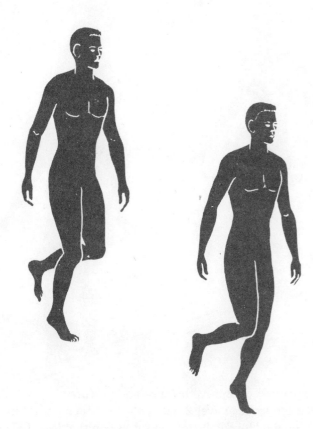

OBJECTIVE: To improve balance, strengthen the extensor muscles of the leg and foot, and increase circulation.

BASIC EXERCISE: Stand erect, lower back flat, with your weight on your right foot and your left leg bent at the knee and your left foot several inches off the floor. Hold your arms slightly outward from your body to aid in balance. Hop five times on your right foot, and then hop five times on your left foot.

EXERCISE 22. KNEE PUSH-UP

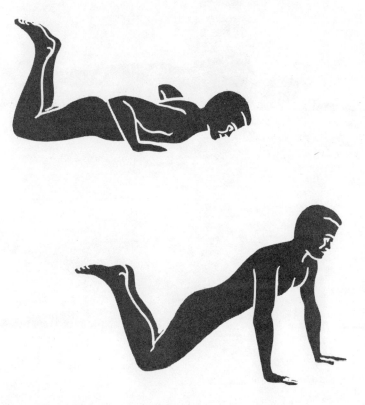

OBJECTIVE: To strengthen the muscles of your arms, shoulders, and trunk.

BASIC EXERCISE: Lie on the floor with your face down, legs together, knees bent, with feet off the floor and your hands palm-down flat on the floor under your shoulders. Slowly push your upper body off the floor, extending your arms fully and keeping your lower back flat so that your body is in a straight line from head to knees. Then slowly return to starting position, then repeat.

EXERCISE 23. SIDE LEG RAISE

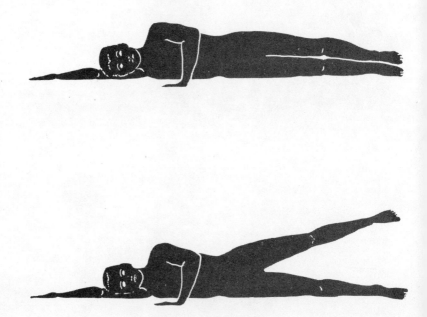

OBJECTIVE: To improve the flexibility of the hip joint and strengthen the lateral muscles of the trunk and hip.

BASIC EXERCISE: Lie on the floor on your right side with your head resting on your right arm and both legs extended together. Lift your extended left leg sideways (upward) off the right leg as far as possible. Stop, then return to the starting position and repeat. After the proper number of repetitions are done with the left leg, roll over on your left side and repeat the exercise with your right leg.

EXERCISE 24. PARTIAL SIT-UP

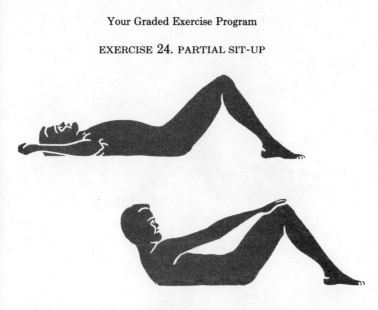

OBJECTIVE: To strengthen lower back and abdominal muscles.

BASIC EXERCISE: Lie on your back on a covered floor with your knees well bent. Squeeze your buttocks and tighten your abdominal muscles, with your lower back on the floor, slowly raise your head, neck, and, last of all, shoulders as you extend your arms to your knees. Keep your lower back flat on the floor. Hold this position ten seconds, then return to starting position, rest a few seconds and repeat. Keep your knees bent. In the beginning it may help to place your feet under a heavy chair or some other restraint. Once your abdominal muscles are strong enough, this should not be necessary and should not be done, since this action actually allows your legs to help the abdomen in allowing you to raise. The motion should be a gentle smooth curling and uncurling. Never jerk to achieve greater height or an additional repetition, and never strain or exert yourself beyond reasonable comfort. Again start with three repetitions and progress to at least ten.

EXERCISE 25. ADVANCED SIT-UP

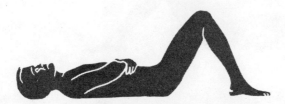

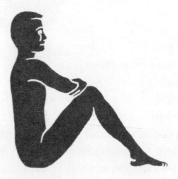

OBJECTIVE: To maximally strengthen lower back and abdominal muscles.

BASIC EXERCISE: Lie on your back on a covered floor with your knees well bent. Squeeze your buttocks and tighten your abdominal muscles. Start with your arms folded over your waist, and smoothly lift your head, shoulders, and back up to a position so that your arms are touching your knees. Hold ten seconds, return to the starting position, relax a few seconds, and then repeat. Again start with three repetitions and progress to at least ten.

EXERCISE 26. ADVANCED MODIFIED SIT-UP

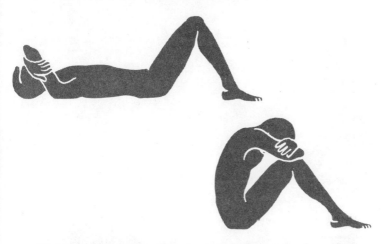

OBJECTIVE: To maximally strengthen lower back and abdominal muscles.

BASIC EXERCISE: Progress gradually until ten of the basic advanced sit-ups can be easily and comfortably executed. Then try folding your arms in front of your face instead of your waist. As you curl up to your knees, hold ten seconds, then return to the starting position, relax a few seconds and repeat. Start with three repetitions. When this modified version can be accomplished ten times, you are ready to attempt a sit-up with your hands clasped behind your head. When this version can also be done ten times, you may, if you wish, attempt the maximal version of a sit-up. This involves lying on your back on a padded inclined surface (i.e., a tilt board with the foot end elevated). Knees should be bent as always; then, with hands clasped behind your neck, slowly and carefully execute the sit-up, hold ten seconds, slowly uncurl to the starting position, relax, and repeat. This last version is clearly optional. The more inclined the board, the greater strength and effort will be required of your back and abdomen to accomplish the sit-up.

EXERCISE 27. SITTING BEND

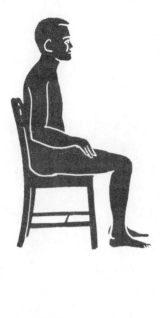

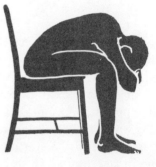

OBJECTIVE: To strengthen your lower back while stretching your lower back and hamstring muscles.

BASIC EXERCISE: Sit on a hard chair, feet flat on the floor, knees not more than 12 inches apart, arms folded loosely in your lap. Squeeze buttocks and tighten abdominal muscles so that your back is flat against the chair. Bend over, letting your head go between your knees, with your hands reaching for the floor. Bend as far as is comfortable, hold for a count of five, then slowly pull your body back to the starting position with your back flat against the chair. Relax a few seconds, then repeat initially three times, gradually increasing to ten repetitions.

EXERCISE 28. DIVER'S STANCE

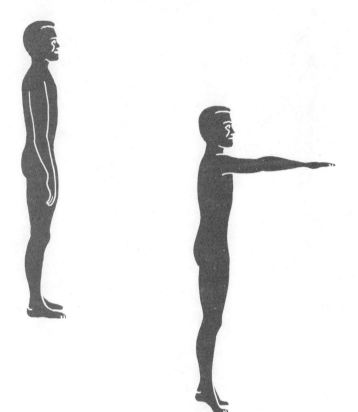

OBJECTIVE: To improve balance and posture while strengthening extensor muscles of the legs and feet.

BASIC EXERCISE: Stand erect with your buttocks and abdomen tensed, feet slightly apart, and your arms at your sides. Lift up on your toes while holding your arms upward and forward so they are extended, palms down at shoulder height, parallel to the floor. Hold this position for ten seconds then return to the starting position and repeat.

EXERCISE 29. DEEP KNEE BEND

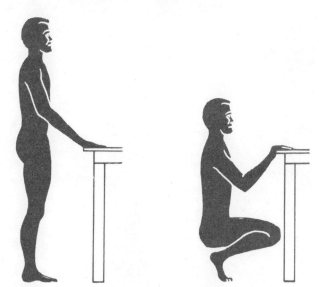

OBJECTIVE: To strengthen the hamstrings and quadriceps muscles.

CAUTION: Do not begin this exercise until you can do a good Back Flattener. Have someone confirm that you are indeed holding your back flat while executing Exercise 6. Most people should not attempt this exercise until a month into this exercise program. Discontinue this exercise if there is considerable lasting discomfort in your knees or hips, and do not try it if you have a history of knee problems.

BASIC EXERCISE: Stand behind a sofa, desk, or heavy chair, holding onto it for balance. Squeeze and tighten your buttocks and abdomen. Slowly bend your knees and, with a flat back, squat down as far as is reasonably comfortable; stop, then stand up using only your legs and not your arms. Relax for a second or two and then repeat, initially three times, gradually building up to ten repetitions.

Then, to complete the sequence, repeat Exercise 2, the Alternate Walk-Jog, with the following modifications:

BASIC EXERCISE: Level 1: Gradually increase to walk 100 steps, then jog 100 steps, alternately for 5 minutes.

Level 2: Walk 50 steps, then jog 25 steps, alternately for 3 to 6 minutes.

Level 3: Walk 50 steps, then jog 10 steps, alternately for 1 to 3 minutes.

And finish with Exercise 1, the Walk.

6.
Special Tips for the Exercising Diabetic

HOW TO PREPARE FOR VIGOROUS EXERCISE

In preparing for vigorous exercise, the insulin-dependent diabetic must be aware of certain conditions that significantly lower sugar levels. For example, the hypoglycemic effect produced by exercise is aggravated by a thigh injection in an exercising leg and should be avoided. Also, either extremely hot or cold weather causes the body to work harder and expend more energy (burn more glucose) to maintain its thermostatic status quo. Exercising into a wind has a similar effect. The same is true of virus colds or other infections. In women diabetics, the menstrual period and pregnancy require greater energy and, coupled with exercise, can profoundly lower the sugar level. In these situations, the diabetic can make one of two adjustments: Decrease insulin or increase caloric intake. For diabetics exercising for health, both a reduction of insulin and a moderate increase of readily usable carbohydrate immediately before exercise will strike an ideal balance. For the competitive athlete, maximal performance is achieved when insulin is left unchanged and considerable carbohydrate is ingested just prior to the competition. In following this prescription, Bobby Clark, a superstar in professional hockey, explains, "I tried to change insulin doses to help with control, but I found it was easier for me to change my food intake to conform with my changing level of activity." To avoid an insulin reaction during competition, some diabetics try for a slight spill as they begin their exercise. For example, Bill Talbert, the tennis player, states, "I try to be slightly on the plus side and stay there during my exercise." This is the same approach taken by hockey star Bobby Clark. By trial and error these athletes discovered the medical fact that performance is impaired by hypoglycemia. Thus, for maximal performance, the diabetic should ingest carbohydrate prior to and during vigorous exercise.

If the diabetic is to avoid hypoglycemia during exercise, he must start it with either a mildly elevated blood sugar level or some rapidly absorbable carbohydrate in his stomach. However, let me caution that the opposite condition, high blood sugar, will also undermine sports proficiency, not to mention long-term health. While a slight rise in blood sugar before vigorous exercise will improve performance and prevent an insulin reaction, too much can be ruinous. Some acceptable preexercise foods that combine short-term (concentrated sugar) and long-term (slower-acting carbohydrates and proteins) energy are:

Apples	Graham crackers
Bananas	Junior baby foods
Beef jerky	Maple sugar candy
Breakfast squares	Milk
Cheese and crackers	Nuts, especially peanuts
Chocolate-covered wafers	Peanut butter crackers
Cookies	Potato chips
Cupcakes	Raisins
Dried fruit	Sweet rolls
Doughnuts (plain)	Various sandwiches

When you are strenuously exercising, it is only safe to err on the side of too much carbohydrate. Most of the diabetic marathoners I interviewed in 1979 were exercising daily and did not change their usual insulin dose unless exercise had to be skipped, in which case most took 15 percent to 25 percent more insulin. As one marathoner, Professor Edward Leete, said, "I do not attempt to change my insulin dosage. If I run for longer distances, I will simply increase my carbohydrate intake." Although this works fine for Professor Leete, if the exercise is more than twice the daily norm, many will want to reduce the insulin intake as well. Whether it be the usual daily workout or a longer run, each runner I talked with echoed the sentiments of marathoner Mike McNally: "Special preparation is essential. Nothing can be left to chance." Preexercise preparation includes (for the nondiabetic as well) consumption of considerable quantities of fluids. When possible, you should ingest an amount of fluid roughly approximate to the anticipated loss. Besides water, beverages like coffee, fruit juice, Coke and other soft drinks, and even Tang and Gatorade are acceptable. None of the diabetic runners I spoke with espoused the currently popular preference for beer as their preexercise fluid supplement, an acceptable but hardly ideal fluid in this case. While care is taken to drink fluids prior to a workout, all diabetic runners also make provisions to have fluids available during the run. Some carry a plastic water bottle or have friends meet them en route with fluids; others actually plan the run according to available sources of fluids—parks, gas stations, or grocery stores.

If your activity is cross-country or downhill skiing, rock climbing, or just hiking, you will have to bring your carbohydrate and fluid source with you. If you exert yourself continuously, I recommend you ingest both a small amount of carbohydrate and water equal to sweat loss each hour. Although they may eat a small amount of food hourly, if they continuously exercise, most diabetics will have negative urines at the day's end.

A second necessary preparation, besides the consumption of carbohydrates before exercising, is the provision for carrying some sugar with you while you exercise. Again, preferences range from sugar cubes to candy bars to fruit slices. Many diabetic runners carry their lunches in a plastic bag so that sweat or splashed water will not spoil them. Marathoner Jim Thacker described his excellent arrangement: "I now wear a belt with an attached pocket around my waist—it has a small plastic bottle and several pockets that will hold sugar, candy, etc. For diabetic runners, it is about perfect." I might add that such an arrangement would be especially suitable for the diabetic bicyclist, canoer, or skier.

Additional preexercise suggestions include making certain that your running partners or a friend know what your route is, and when to expect you back. Marathoner Bill Royston adds: "When running a very long distance, fifteen miles and up, I carry emergency money and have the route of the run pass near convenience stores or gas stations, particularly near the end of the run."

HOW TO HANDLE AN INSULIN REACTION WHILE EXERCISING

For most diabetics, an insulin reaction begins with a light-headed, dizzy sensation and is followed by a feeling of weakness, palpitations, and cold, clammy skin. Individual symptoms can vary markedly. For some, personality changes may even occur, with a belligerent, ill-tempered demeanor being not uncommon. Marathoner Tom McManus, Jr., described the onset of a reaction while running as "a scary occurrence. I am awake enough to realize I can't put one foot in front of the other. I start landing on pointed toes. In retrospect, the prospect of death was never as imminent as the incapacitation of my legs, which were uncontrollable." While somewhat dramatic, his comment does emphasize diminishing coordination, which is one of the very first signs of hypoglycemia in an exercising diabetic.

Most diabetics quickly learn to read their own signals of low blood sugar. If you are exercising when the signals arrive stop immediately and drink a quick-acting sugary beverage, such as orange juice, or eat honey or a candy bar. "The point is," said runner Bill Royston, "each of us needs to learn our exercise limitations, how long we can go without refueling our sugar supply, and be close to a sugar source when a hypoglycemic reaction does occur." It is imperative that you act promptly because mental judgment is one of the first faculties to go in an insulin reaction. The most efficient remedy is sugar already dissolved in fluid; however, sugar usually acts rapidly enough when eaten. No exercising diabetic should ever be without an emergency sugar supply. Lifesavers are handy and efficient and enter the bloodstream even faster than sugar because they contain corn syrup, a form of glucose. Not recommended are chocolate candy bars, because they are messy and act slower than other candies because of their relatively high fat content.

How much sugar is enough? This, of course, is not a constant, since each occurrence may have multiple precipitating factors and vary in severity. However, guidelines do exist, and for most diabetics 10 to 15 grams of glucose are sufficient to reverse a reaction. In its Diabetes Teaching Guide, the Joslin Clinic advises: "Treat all reactions immediately. Take a simple, fast-acting sugar and allow it to have ten to fifteen minutes to act. Repeat the same dose of sugar if no improvement with the first."

The amount of sugar that the exercising diabetic carries with him does not have to be absolutely precise. Actually a couple of rolls of hard candy or half a dozen sugar cubes in most instances do the trick nicely. Typical sugar contents of some commonly available foods are:

Corn syrup (Karo)	1 tablespoon = 15 grams
Cube sugar	2 cubes = 12 grams
Honey	1 tablespoon = 16 grams
Jam	1 teaspoon = 14 grams
Jelly	1 teaspoon = 13 grams
Lifesavers	3 candies = 10 grams
Maple syrup	1 tablespoon = 13 grams
Orange juice	½ cup = 10 grams
Sugar	2 packets (2 teaspoons) = 8 grams
Sweetened soda pop	½ cup = 20 grams

If you have no sugar—something the diabetic, and particularly the exercising diabetic, should never be without—then send a companion for some while you lie down, relaxed and motionless, to expend as little energy as possible. This is why common sense dictates that the diabetic should never exercise alone and that his or her companion should be able to treat a reaction. It is tempting to exercise alone especially when running or jogging. Yet although some diabetics have accomplished incredible feats alone, it is just not sensible.

The diabetic should be aware of the times of the day when an insulin reaction is most likely to occur, based on when insulin was taken and what type was used. Today almost all diabetics use either NPH or regular insulin. Since NPH is longer acting, with a peak action of six to ten hours after injection but a total duration of effect of sixteen to twenty-four hours, it is usually given only in the morning. This necessitates that you eat a hearty lunch, if vigorous exercise is pursued in the early to mid-afternoon. Regular insulin with a peak effect two to three hours after injection and a duration of six to eight hours, is usually used as a supplemental dose before the evening meal. But, for some, it is the sole source of insulin and must be administered before every meal. Professor Edward Leete explained: "After much trial and error, I was able to achieve control with injections of regular insulin before each meal. I currently take fifteen units before breakfast, ten units before lunch [he runs daily after the noon meal], and fifteen units before dinner."

A special word of caution should be mentioned with regard to the diabetic who runs late in the day or has burned up more calories than usual but has eaten a light dinner. The NPH insulin injected at 7 A.M. is still active long after midnight. If a late snack of a slowly metabolized carbohydrate or protein is not ingested, a nocturnal insulin reaction may occur. This can be especially unfortunate because, since the diabetic is asleep, he has no chance to ward off the reaction. Since each moderate to severe insulin reaction can be equated with a brain concussion, this repeated trauma to your brain is to be avoided, even at the cost of occasionally spilling some sugar. It is far less injurious to be a bit hyperglycemic than to have a hypoglycemic reaction, especially a nocturnal one.

The diabetic is encouraged by the medical profession to wear a Medic Alert bracelet with the information that he is a diabetic taking insulin. Despite the medical sophistication of the public today, I still find the suggestion of marathoner Jim Thacker meritorious. Instead of having just *diabetes* on your bracelet or identification card, he suggests you add *give me sugar* to leave no doubt as to what you need if you are found to be not in control of your mental faculties.

WHERE TO INJECT YOUR INSULIN

Most diabetics have been instructed to rotate the insulin injection sites, using both upper arms, thighs, buttocks, and sides of the abdomen. A common practice is to give each injection in a straight horizontal line about one inch apart. After finishing a straight line with four or five injections, move to the next arm, leg, buttock, or side of the abdomen. When a full rotation has been completed, return to the original line and drop down one inch and repeat. After four or five lines, which usually represents an equal number of months, return to the original line.

One problem that a physical fitness program poses for the diabetic is that exercise can increase the rate of insulin absorption, depending upon the site of administration. The exact mechanism for increased insulin absorption is uncertain, but apparently it is related to the increased blood flow to the area affected by the exercise. Thus, leg exercise has been shown to increase the rate of absorption of insulin subcutaneously injected into the thigh or buttock. Because of this tendency, the diabetic is cautioned to use a nonexercised site for his or her insulin injection. If you do not you significantly increase the risk of a hypoglycemic reaction.

Although diabetics can inject insulin subcutaneously anywhere in the body, recent studies indicate that exercise has no effect on the absorption of insulin from the arm or abdominal wall. In fact, in these studies the disappearance of insulin from the abdominal wall was slightly retarded in the postexercise period. Therefore, for most exercises that require movement of both the upper and lower body, the abdominal wall is the preferred site for an injection that precedes vigorous exercise. (See Figure 3.) For the runner it appears that either the arm or abdominal wall is adequate. This usually means the morning injection, if the exercise is to be done during the day. The arm, thigh, and buttock can be used for the evening insulin postexercise injection, if a second dose is taken. But if exercise is to be done at night, both the morning and evening insulin injections should be given in the abdominal site.

MUST INSULIN ALWAYS BE KEPT REFRIGERATED?

The notion that the insulin itself must be kept refrigerated poses an awkward and unnecessary problem for the diabetic.

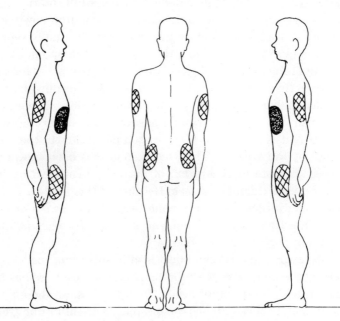

Fig. 3. Recommended Insulin Injection Sites
Before ▨ and After ▧ Exercise

Unless one stays at home, the constant refrigeration of insulin
becomes difficult, if not downright impossible, especially for diabetics using multiple daily administrations of insulin. In reality, you need not worry about the potency of your insulin unless you freeze it, which ruins it, or subject it to very high
temperatures, which weakens it. If you are outside in the winter cold skiing, simply keep it in a packet close to your body.
When traveling in the heat, merely keep it out of direct sun-
light. Of course, when refrigeration is available, use it. But realize that insulin will retain its potency at room temperature for
days—and some have claimed even up to a year.

SKIN INFECTIONS AND THE EXERCISING DIABETIC

One of the fears instilled in many exercising diabetics is that they are highly prone to infection. This has caused almost hysterical concern among some diabetics regarding the consequences of hangnails, ingrown toenails, superficial cuts and abrasions, not to mention common viral colds. In hopes of avoiding these minor problems, some diabetics religiously consume daily quantities of Vitamin C, Vitamin B_{12}, Vitamin E, and the others. This only psychologically benefits the diabetic on a balanced diet. Furthermore, the young and middle-aged diabetic under good control may anticipate healing as rapidly as the nondiabetic and with little more chance of infection.

For the diabetic with more than twenty years of insulin use or at an advanced age, healing may be retarded and the chance of infection enhanced if vascular disease is present. Here, slow healing is a result not of the diabetes but rather of poor circulation. If circulation is inadequate to meet the metabolic demands of the tissues, then healing will be retarded and the chance of infection increased. This is why there are so many oblique references in diabetic material to "foot problems."

While young diabetics should not worry about healing and infection, it is common sense to pay careful attention to any cuts, abrasions, or blisters. This is especially true of the feet, where the affected area is difficult to keep clean. If you do sustain a cut, blister, or other foot injury, immediate attention should be given, resting, soaking, and cleansing the injured area.

Good foot care includes washing daily with soap and warm—never extremely hot—water. The skin should be blotted dry thoroughly, especially between the toes. Once the foot is dry, a lanolin cream will aid in keeping the skin soft, as will an antifungal cream. Toenails should be kept clean; remove dirt with orangewood sticks or cotton swabs and clip the nails square.

If an infection or injury occurs, a supermaximal effort at diabetic control, the strictest avoidance of spilling sugar in the urine, must be made. This cannot be too strongly stressed. It is discouraging to hear some authorities state that half of the young diabetics never experience good control. It is the expressed intent of this book to provide a means of reducing that figure to as near zero as possible for the insulin-dependent diabetic and of preventing the onset of disease in most adult-onset cases.

AN ADVANTAGE IN BEING DIABETIC

Some may ask if I am joking when I imply that there may be advantages in being diabetic. Not at all! Of necessity, diabetics must acquire self-discipline in relation to their own diet, exercise, and, if required, medicine. Of course, this self-discipline carries over into other activities demanding daily determination and stick-to-itiveness, such as sports, school, and work. Mary Tyler Moore has been quoted as saying: "I feel very positive about my 'malfunction.' It means I go to the doctor more than most people and exercise more than most people and watch my diet more than most people. And, as a consequence, I think I'm healthier than most people." The controlled young and middle-aged diabetic often is in better health than his obese, nonexercising, nondiabetic friends whose diets are too high in saturated fat and calories. And since the diabetic has regular physical examinations, other physical problems have an excellent chance of being detected earlier than in the nondiabetic who is likely to have physical checkups more sporadically.

"I looked upon it as a challenge to mold perhaps an even healthier life than before," said runner Mark Collins. And marathoner Mike McNally believes that, as a result of becoming diabetic, "I have a greater appreciation for the human body and life itself."

And since exercise is a vital factor in treating diabetes, the fun of pursuing it can be a major priority in the life of the diabetic. "Diabetes," said marathoner Tom McManus, Jr., "is a major excuse to run. In that sense, diabetes supports my lifestyle, rather than vice versa." While the nondiabetic may skip a set of tennis because he or she feels guilty "having fun" instead of finishing work, the diabetic realizes that exercise is vital to his daily medical treatment and that only by pursuing it can he be at his best at work. Television personality Dan Rowen exercises daily, does body-building calisthenics twice a week, and plays tennis four to six times a week as part of his conditioning program. I dare say, many people would love to have a doctor *prescribe* such recreational pursuits for them.

Marathoner Bill Royston pointed out that "exercise should be planned ahead of time and on a regular basis. If insulin dosage and food consumption are geared for a certain amount of exercise, it is hard to deviate too far from the planned workout without having a deficit or excess of sugar in the system. There are many times when a runner would rather stay in bed than run; however, being diabetic gives me the extra incentive to exercise every day." According to runner Jim Kirk, "The only possible concessions to having diabetes ... I have [made are] that I must be extra cautious about diet, sleep, injuries, and flexibility. All of these are important to the competitive runner, and, as a result of my precautions, I have become a better runner."

Many of the marathoners I spoke with had similar comments. Professor Edward Leete remarks: "My initial reaction was one of annoyance; however, when I realized that I could control myself well with insulin, I became resigned to the situation. I believe that I became a serious athlete, a long-distance runner to prove to myself and others that I could be as fit and healthy as the nondiabetic." Jim Thacker says: "My first question after the diagnosis of diabetes was, can I do what others do? When I found that I could, I moved to the point where I can do more than ninety-nine percent of the population—at least in an endurance sense." John Cass commented: "I believe so completely in endurance exercise for diabetics that I believe a few of us that do it all the time should train new diabetics; not only new diabetics, but diabetics who want to put their bodies and minds in the shape they should be."

7.

Planning the Fit Diabetic's Exercise Program

THE DAILY REGIMEN

As discussed previously, the essence of physical fitness is a fit cardiovascular system. Having attained Level 1 status, as determined in chapter 5, it is now time to liberalize and vary your daily exercise program to make it more stimulating and enjoyable. The rest of this chapter is devoted to showing you how you can do this for yourself. Certain basic concepts, however, should be stressed. For example, your exercise program should include exercises that promote flexibility, coordination, agility, balance, muscular strength, and endurance. Muscles, if not used, grow soft and atrophy. The natural, slow decline of muscular strength and endurance can be retarded only by keeping the muscles toned by means of regular exercise. So too, the balance and equilibrium mechanisms of the body can be kept fit only through use; accelerated degeneration occurs with disuse. The tissue surrounding joints increase in thickness and lose their elasticity with advancing years. As is true in the case of arthritis, this process is greatly retarded by a daily exercise program that moves the joints through the full range of motion.

Exercise will keep your joints flexible, your muscles supple and springy, and your heart feeling young.

To be of maximal benefit, your exercise program should be carried out daily. It should have three parts: a *warm-up period,* an *endurance phase,* and a *cooling-off period.* It is analogous to the racehorse warming up, running the race, and returning to the paddock to be cooled off by walking.

THE WARM-UP PERIOD

The warm-up period should be at least five minutes long and include rhythmic slow stretching movements of the trunk and limb muscles. This increases blood flow and stretches the postural muscles, preparing the body for sustained activity. To ignore the warm-up is to risk muscle pulls or more severe injuries. The list below gives fourteen warm-up exercises. You may choose any combination of three for your five-minute warm-up period. Start with three repetitions and gradually build to ten or more. Vary the combinations on different days to avoid monotony.

1. Back Flattener (Exercise 6)
2. Single Knee Raise (Exercise 13)
3. Single Knee Hug (Exercise 14)
4. Double Knee Hug (Exercise 15)
5. Single Leg Raise (Exercise 16)
6. Partial Sit-up (Exercise 24)
7. Advanced Sit-up (Exercise 25)
8. Sitting Bend (Exercise 27)
9. Deep Knee Bend (Exercise 29)
10. Posture Check (Exercise 8)
11. Bend and Stretch (Exercise 3)
12. Wall Push-up (Exercise 12)
13. Hop 3 minutes (Exercise 21)
14. Diver's Stance (Exercise 28)

THE ENDURANCE PHASE

The endurance phase should last at least fifteen to thirty minutes. During this period your cardiovascular system is stressed to increase aerobic capacity. What are the best cardiovascular exercises for you? It has been said that the best exercise is the one you most enjoy because it is the one you will most likely continue to do. Certain characteristics are most desirable and, thus, make some exercises more beneficial than others.

First, from a cardiovascular standpoint, the primary objective is sustained vigorous exercise pursued for a length of time sufficient to burn in excess of 400 calories. By sustained is meant that the exercise must be done continuously without stopping. If you plan to exercise for thirty or more minutes, do not stop once during that period of time. Already you can guess that sports such as football, with a huddle between every play, rank low as a fitness exercise pursuit. The activity should increase your heart rate to approximately 75 percent to 80 percent of its maximal potential in order for you to experience cardiovascular improvement. For most of us, this translates into a pulse rate of around 120 to 150 beats per minutes to achieve this increased endurance fitness. Practically speaking, this also translates into a 75 percent to 80 percent maximal oxygen consumption. To exceed 80 percent of maximal cardiac output as measured by pulse rate may lead to inadequate oxygenation; that is, you cannot consume oxygen fast enough, so your body shifts to anaerobic or nonoxygen metabolism, which may cause tissue damage. In reality, most exercise is achieved at a lower pulse rate.

Another feature of endurance involves the ability to increase the workload as your level of fitness increases. With increased fitness, the same activity that initially caused a pulse rate of 140 may now produce an increase to only 100. Thus, the activity must be made progressively more difficult. This can be accomplished in one of two ways. You can slowly increase the overall rate at which you carry out the exercise. The progress should be accomplished in many small steps. Or you can introduce intervals of a faster pace alternating with a slower pace. The faster pace should be sufficiently vigorous so that you incur an oxygen debt; then switch to a slower pace in order to replenish your oxygen debt. Competitive athletes use interval training extensively, but you will probably prefer to increase your pace slowly at a comfortable rate as your fitness progresses.

Tables 4, 5, and 6 classify sports as heavy, moderate, or light-moderate, according to their exercise value and the energy output they require. A number of household projects are also graded and can be substituted in the exercise program as endurance activities. In the heavy exercise group, these include chopping wood, shoveling snow, and digging holes; in the moderate group, scrubbing floors and performing heavy gardening chores like mowing the lawn or pulling weeds; in the light-moderate group, sweeping floors, ironing, washing clothes, making beds, and doing light work in the garden.

A few comments on the relative merits and demerits of various activities seem appropriate to this discussion. In my opinion, the finest three activities for total body conditioning are swimming, cross-country skiing, and roller skiing. Unlike jogging, which does little to strengthen or increase upper-body joint flexibility, each of these three combines a vigorous cardiovascular endurance workout with strengthening and increased flexibility of all the joints. On the negative side, swimming is boring for many, cross-country skiing requires snow, and roller skiing does subject one to the risks of falling.

The second tier of ideal sports for conditioning (the heavy exercise group) includes jogging, cycling, rope skipping, and rowing. Jogging and rope skipping are the least expensive and most expedient. Cycling and rowing may each involve an expensive initial outlay of money, and cycling, if practiced on city streets, can be dangerous. But the great advantage of this fit-

TABLE 4
ENERGY EXPENDITURES FOR LIGHT-MODERATE ACTIVITIES

RECREATIONAL ACTIVITIES

(200–400 calories burned/hour)

Archery*	Croquet*	Horseback riding*	Shuffleboard*
Baseball	Fishing*	Horseshoes*†	Walking
Bowling*†	Golf*	Sailing*	(~5mph on level)*

HOUSEHOLD ACTIVITIES

(1–3 calories per minute for a 150-pound person. To be used as an endurance workout these activities must be pursued very vigorously in a nonstop manner for 1½–2 hours.)

Making the bed	Making minor repairs on the car
Cleaning the tub	Building with wood
Ironing clothes	Painting
Putting away groceries	Shampooing rugs with an electric cleaner
Vacuuming the floor or pool	
Dusting	Walking on a level or downhill surface
Washing clothes by hand	
Washing floors, walls, or windows	Raking leaves
	Paperhanging
Light gardening	Bricklaying
Mowing the lawn with a power mower	Cleaning windows
	Light carpentry
Pruning bushes	Janitorial work
Cutting hedges with an electric cutter	Sewing, knitting
	Playing a musical instrument
Washing or waxing the car by hand	

* Recommended for persons over fifty by the International Committee on the Standardization of Physical Fitness.
† Should be approached cautiously by those with back problems.

TABLE 5
ENERGY EXPENDITURES FOR MODERATE ACTIVITIES

RECREATIONAL ACTIVITIES

(400–600 calories burned/hour)

Badminton*	Curling*	Skating*	Touch football
Baseball	Dancing*	Skindiving	Volleyball*
Bicycling	Deck tennis*	Softball	Water skiing†
(~10mph)*	Fencing	Squash	
Canoeing*	Paddle tennis*	Table tennis*	
Cricket	Rowing*	Tennis*†	

HOUSEHOLD ACTIVITIES

(4–6 calories per minute for a 150-pound person. To be used as an endurance workout these activities must be pursued very vigorously in a nonstop manner for 60–75 minutes.)

Mowing the lawn with a hand mower	Walking up small hills
Hoeing	Walking in water
Spading the garden	Walking in loose sand on a level
Raking leaves	Pushing a loaded wheelbarrow
Pulling weeds	Carrying 30–50 pounds on a level
Playing a musical instrument energetically	Painting requiring a ladder
Sawing wood by hand	Cutting hedges with hand clipper
Splitting logs by hand	Sanding wood, metal, etc.
Vigorously mopping or scrubbing floors	Light-moderate activities done vigorously

---

* Recommended for persons over fifty by the International Committee on the Standardization of Physical Fitness.
† Should be approached cautiously by those with back problems.

---

ness program is that you can tailor it to your own likes and dislikes. Practically any vigorous physical activity can be used in the endurance phase, provided it is performed for a long enough period of time and with sufficient intensity. For example, a weekend ski trip or a vigorous tennis match can count for

TABLE 6
ENERGY EXPENDITURES FOR HEAVY ACTIVITIES

RECREATIONAL ACTIVITIES

(600–900 calories burned/hour)

Bicycling (10mph uphill)*	Mountain climbing
Cross-country skiing	Roller Skiing
Deep-sea fishing (with fish on)*	Rugby
Handball	Swimming*
Jogging†	

HOUSEHOLD ACTIVITIES

(7–10 calories per minute for a 150-pound person. To be used as an endurance workout these activities must be pursued very vigorously in a nonstop manner for 30 45 minutes.)

Chopping wood	Shoveling dirt, sand, manure,
Digging holes	etc.
Shoveling snow	Carrying anything over 50
Walking up steep hills	pounds
Walking up stairs	Moderate activities done vig-
Carrying 30–50 pounds up an	orously so as to produce a
incline	heart rate of 120–130 beats
	per minute

* Recommended for persons over fifty by the International Committee for the Standardization of Physical Fitness.
† Should be approached cautiously by those with back problems.

one of the required workouts. Or you can substitute hard physical labor, like snow shoveling or sawing wood, for one of the endurance periods. If you enjoy sports, then you can substitute on any given day thirty minutes of maximal exercise sports, i.e., running, stationary running, cycling, cross-country skiing, or swimming; sixty minutes of moderate sports activity, i.e., tennis, skiing, etc.; or ninety minutes of minimal exercise sports, i.e., golf, gardening, canoeing, bowling, fishing, archery, horseshoes, Ping-Pong, shuffleboard, or social dancing. The time periods, of course, can be of any desired duration.

Whichever exercise you select from the tables, the primary emphasis should be on *safe* and *enjoyable* participation. Since few will adhere to an exercise commitment that is not pleasurable, it is best to do whatever you most enjoy. On those days when the weather is poor outside or when you cannot exercise in daylight, you may substitute if necessary the indoor activities of jogging in place, walking stairs, rope skipping, stationary bicycle riding, etc.

THE COOLING-OFF PERIOD

The cooling-off period is too often omitted in exercise programs. Whereas the endurance phase significantly raises body temperature, increases the heart rate and blood pressure, and builds up lactic acid and other waste products in your muscles, the cooling-off phase allows the bodily functions to gradually return to normal and it helps to eliminate waste products from your muscles, minimizing the chance of stiffness and soreness the next day. The cooling-off phase should last at least five minutes and can last longer if you want it to. It should include large body movements that emphasize the range of motion of the joints. Calisthenics are ideal for this final step in your day's exercise program. I would recommend that you select any three exercises from the following list; start with three repetitions and build to at least ten. As with the warm-ups, vary your selection to avoid boredeom.

1. Walk 5 minutes (Exercise 1)
2. Alternate Walk-Jog 3 minutes (Exercise 2)
3. Rotate Head (Exercise 4)
4. Body Bender (Exercise 5)
5. Wall Press (Exercise 7)
6. Arm Circles (Exercise 9)
7. Half Knee Bend (Exercise 10)

8. Wing Stretcher (Exercise 11)
9. Single Leg Raise and Knee Hug (Exercise 17)
10. Straight Arm and Leg Stretch (Exercise 18)
11. Heel-Toe Walk (Exercise 19)
12. Heel-Toe Beam Walk (Exercise 20)
13. Knee Push-up (Exercise 22)
14. Side Leg Raise (Exercise 23)

FOR THE SUPER ACHIEVER

Inevitably, some people, having attained Level 1 fitness, will seek even more vigorous endurance activity, such as the extremes of our diabetic marathoners. Although this is to be applauded, I caution you not to substitute jogging for your entire exercise program. A splendid cardiovascular exercise, it does little for your upper-body muscle tone or joint flexibility and mobility. Therefore, jogging should always be preceded by stretching and followed by the cooling-off exercises.

Several additional points on jogging are especially pertinent to the diabetic, who should be especially cognizant of proper foot hygiene. First, if you jog, you *must* wear appropriate running shoes. Basketball shoes, sneakers, or deck shoes will not suffice. Specially constructed running shoes provide foot and arch support and have multilayered flat nonskid soles that cushion the force of impact as you land on your feet. Unlike tennis shoes, which do not have widths, good running shoes come in a variety of widths, and extreme care is essential in obtaining a precise fit. Most podiatrists recommend trying on shoes at the end of the day when your feet have swollen to their maximum size.

In addition, when jogging, wear soft, loose-fitting clothing. Tight-fitting or abrasive clothing, heavy from perspiration, will chafe the skin, especially the nipples, groin, and armpits. It is seldom too cold to jog if you wear adequate clothing, gloves, and a hat or cap with adequate ear protection. Only a low wind-chill factor should force you to exercise indoors, since jogging then may result in frostbite.

Also, never jog on ice or other slippery surfaces.

While it is rarely too cold to jog in winter, in summer it is often too hot. Do not jog at midday, especially when temperatures and humidity are high. And replenish lost body fluids promptly either during or after your warm weather workout.

Nighttime jogging is also dangerous because you may stumble and fall. Only if a running area is adequately illuminated, for example, at a lighted track, or if you wear a headlight, should you jog at night, and then only over known flat surfaces.

Finally, let me again state the risks of competing in sports as opposed to following a personal fitness program. *Competition should be avoided if the primary objective is only physical fitness because competition will invariably bring with it a stress-related injury resulting in an enforced layoff.* The injury rate for the competitive athlete nears 100 percent. However, for some people, it is the stimulus of competition that makes otherwise tedious exercise more tolerable. Training that is not directed toward a specific objective is difficult to maintain. A more individualized approach to sports is an ideal compromise. In distance races, for example, so many people usually enter that except for three or four in each class, the remainder are running against their own previous best time, certainly a more controlled and reasonable form of competition, but one that can still be satisfying. If you retain the common sense never to extend yourself too far in competition, the rewards will overshadow any minor injuries you may incur. However, participation in one sport, no matter how vigorous, can never replace a total exercise program.

Finally, I would like to repeat the words of Dr. Fred W. Whitehouse, past president of the American Diabetes Association: "It is clear that the healthiest diabetics are those who are trim and active." Over thirty physiological and emotional benefits accrue to those who exercise regularly. For the diabetic, exercise and proper diet take on even added significance as they enhance the effectiveness of circulating insulin and lower harmful blood fats. This results in the elimination of diabetes in most adult-onset noninsulin-dependent diabetics, and leads to the best possible control and avoidance of complications in both insulin- and noninsulin-dependent diabetics alike. It is not too late. Today is as good a day to begin as any. Let's get started with your diabetic diet and exercise program!

Appendix I
Food Exchanges

MILK EXCHANGES

A single milk contains 12 grams of carbohydrate, 8 grams of protein, a trace of fat and 80 calories. This list demonstrates the kinds and amounts of milk or milk products used for a single milk exchange.

NONFAT FORTIFIED MILK

Skim or nonfat milk	1 cup
Powdered	
(nonfat dry, before adding liquid)	⅓ cup
Canned, evaporated—skim milk	½ cup
Buttermilk made from skim milk	1 cup
Yogurt made from skim milk	
(plain, unflavored)	1 cup

LOW-FAT FORTIFIED MILK

1% fat fortified milk	
(omit ½ fat exchange)	1 cup

2% fat fortified milk	
(omit 1 fat exchange)	1 cup
Yogurt made from 2% fortified milk	
(plain, unflavored)	
(omit 1 fat exchange)	1 cup

WHOLE MILK (OMIT 2 FAT EXCHANGES)

Whole milk	1 cup
Canned, evaporated whole milk	½ cup
Buttermilk made from whole milk	1 cup
Yogurt made from whole milk	
(plain, unflavored)	1 cup

If you want to make a substitution in the milk called for in your diet plan, either choose a milk product that contains the same number of fat exchanges or allow for the difference in your meal plan. For example, if your diet calls for 1 cup of 2 percent milk (1 fat exchange), you may substitute 1 cup of buttermilk (no fat) plus one additional fat exchange.

VEGETABLE EXCHANGES

A single vegetable exchange contains about 5 grams of carbohydrate, 2 grams of protein, and 25 calories. This second list shows kinds of *vegetables* that can be used in a single vegetable exchange. One exchange is ½ cup. (Starchy vegetables are found in the bread exchange list.)

Asparagus	Cabbage	Green pepper
Bean sprouts	Carrots	Greens
Beets	Cauliflower	Beet
Broccoli	Celery	Chard
Brussels	Cucumbers	Collard
sprouts	Eggplant	Dandelion

Kale	Rhubarb	Tomatoes
Mustard	Rutabaga	Tomato juice
Spinach	Sauerkraut	Turnips
Turnip	String beans,	Vegetable juice
Mushrooms	green or yellow	cocktail
Okra	Summer squash	Zucchini
Onions		

The following raw vegetables may be used as desired because they contain so few calories.

Chicory	Endive	Parsley
Chinese	Escarole	Radishes
cabbage	Lettuce	Watercress

These vegetables can also be ordered in a restaurant, but you should try to avoid creamed, scalloped, au gratin, fried, or sautéed vegetables in a sauce. Simply explain to your waiter that you want your vegetables to be raw, steamed, boiled, or plain, with no sauces.

FRUIT EXCHANGES

A single fruit exchange contains 10 grams of carbohydrate and 40 calories.

This third list shows the kinds and amounts of *fruits* to use for a single fruit exchange.

Apple	1 small
Apple juice or cider	⅓ cup
Applesauce (unsweetened)	½ cup
Apricots, fresh	2 medium

Apricots, dried	4	halves
Banana	½	small
Berries:		
Blackberries	½	cup
Blueberries	½	cup
Raspberries	½	cup
Strawberries	¾	cup
Cherries	10	large
Dates	2	
Figs, fresh	1	
Figs, dried	1	
Grapefruit	½	
Grapefruit juice	½	cup
Grapes	12	
Grape juice	¼	cup
Mango	½	small
Melons		
Cantaloupe	¼	small
Honeydew	⅛	medium
Watermelon	1	cup
Nectarine	1	small
Orange	1	small
Orange juice	½	cup
Papaya (fruit)	¾	cup
Peach	1	medium
Pear	1	small
Persimmon, native	1	medium
Pineapple	½	cup
Pineapple juice	⅓	cup
Plums	2	medium
Prunes	2	medium
Prune juice	¼	cup
Raisins	2	tablespoons
Tangerine	1	medium

You may order any fresh fruit while dining, but try to avoid canned fruit, which is usually packed with sugar. The juice-packed fruits are sometimes very popular. They do not have sugar, but they do have more calories than either water-packed or artificially sweetened fruits. You always have to figure the calories in the juice into your diet. If you feel like eating extra without violating the rules of the diet, you may eat cranberries as desired—as long as no sugar is added.

BREAD EXCHANGES

A single bread exchange contains 15 grams of carbohydrate, 2 grams of protein, and 70 calories. Starchy vegetables are included here because they contain, per exchange, the same carbohydrate and protein as one slice of bread. This list shows the kinds and amounts of breads, cereals, and starchy vegetables— as well as prepared foods—to use for a single bread exchange. The prepared foods listed contain fat, so omit one fat exchange when using them.

BREADS

Bagel, small	½	
White (including French and Italian)	1	1-inch slice
Whole wheat	1	1-inch slice
Pumpernickel or rye	1	1-inch slice
Raisin	1	1-inch slice
Dried bread crumbs	3	tablespoons
English muffin, small	½	
Frankfurter roll	½	
Hamburger bun	½	
Plain roll, bread	1	
Tortilla	1	6-inch diam.

CEREALS

Bran flakes	½ cup
Other ready-to-eat, unsweetened cereal	⅓ cup
Cereal puffed (unfrosted)	1 cup
Cereal (cooked)	½ cup
Cornmeal (dry)	2 tablespoons
Flour	2½ tablespoons
Grits (cooked)	½ cup
Pasta (cooked)	½ cup
Popcorn (popped, no fat added)	3 cups
Rice or barley (cooked)	½ cup
Wheat germ	¼ cup

CRACKERS

Arrowroot	3	
Graham	2	2½-inch
Matzo	½	4 × 6-inch
Oyster	20	
Pretzels	25	3⅛ × ⅛-inch
Rye wafers	3	2 × 3½-inch
Saltines	6	
Soda	4	2½-inch

STARCHY VEGETABLES

Beans, peas, lentils (dried and cooked)	½ cup
Baked beans, no pork (canned)	¼ cup
Corn	⅓ cup
Corn on cob	1 small
Lima beans	½ cup
Parsnips	⅔ cup

Peas, green (fresh, canned, or frozen)	½ cup
Potato, white	1 small
Potato, mashed	½ cup
Pumpkin	¾ cup
Winter, acorn, or butternut squash	½ cup
Yam or sweet potato	¼ cup

PREPARED FOODS

Biscuit	1 2-inch diam.
Corn bread	1 2 × 2 × 1-inch
Corn muffin	1 2-inch diam.
Crackers, round butter type	5
Muffin, plain small	1
Pancake	1 5 × ½-inch
Potatoes, french fried	8 2–3½-inch
Potato or corn chips	15
Waffle	1 5 × ½-inch

Breads can be kept track of very easily by their size. When you eat out, white, rye, and whole wheat breads are satisfactory, along with such items as hard and soft rolls, muffins, biscuits, crackers, and English muffins. Go ahead and order those sweet potatoes also.

MEAT EXCHANGES

To plan a diet low in saturated fat and cholesterol, choose only exchanges under "Lean Meats."

LEAN MEATS

One exchange of lean meat (1 ounce) contains 7 grams of protein, 3 grams of fat, and 55 calories. This list shows the kinds and amounts of lean meat and other protein-rich foods to use for a single low-fat meat exchange.

Beef: baby beef (very lean), chipped beef, chuck flank steak, tenderloin plate ribs, plate skirt steak, round (bottom, top), rump (all cuts), spare ribs, tripe	1 ounce
Lamb: leg, rib, sirloin, loin, (roast and chops), shank, shoulder	1 ounce
Pork: leg (whole rump, center shank), smoked ham (center slices)	1 ounce
Poultry: meat (without skin) of chicken, turkey, cornish hen, guinea hen, pheasant	1 ounce
Veal: leg, loin, rib, shank, shoulder, cutlets	1 ounce
Fish: any (fresh or frozen)	1 ounce
canned salmon, tuna, mackerel, crab, and lobster	¼ cup
clams, oysters, scallops, shrimp	5 or 1 ounce
sardines (drained)	3
Other protein sources:	
Cheeses containing less than 5% butterfat	1 ounce
Cottage cheese, dry and 2% butterfat	¼ cup
Dried beans and peas (omit 1 bread exchange)	½ cup

MEDIUM-FAT MEATS

For each exchange of medium-fat meat you eat, omit ½ fat exchange. Each exchange includes 7 grams protein, 5.5 grams fat, and 77 calories. This list shows the kinds and amounts of medium-fat meat and other protein-rich foods to use for one medium-fat meat exchange.

Beef: ground round (15% fat), corned beef (canned), rib-eye	1 ounce
Variety meats: liver, heart, kidneys, and sweetbreads (these are high in cholesterol)	1 ounce
Pork: loin (all cuts tenderloin), shoulder arm (picnic), shoulder blade, boston butt, canadian bacon, boiled ham	1 ounce
Other protein sources:	
Cheese: mozzarella, ricotta, farmer's cheese, Neufchatel	1 ounce
Parmesan	3 tablespoons
Cottage cheese, creamed	¼ cup
Eggs (high in cholesterol)	1
Peanut butter (omit 2 additional fat exchanges)	2 tablespoons

HIGH-FAT MEATS

For each exchange of high-fat meat you eat, omit 1 fat exchange. Each exchange includes 7 grams protein, 8 grams fat, and 100 calories. This list shows the kinds and amounts of high-fat meat and other protein-rich foods to use for one high-fat meat exchange.

Beef: brisket, corned beef brisket, ground chuck (more than 20% fat), roasts (rib) steaks (club and rib)	1 ounce
Cold cuts	1 4½ × ⅛-inch slice
Frankfurter	1 regular
Lamb: breast	1 ounce
Pork: spare ribs, loin (back ribs), ground pork, country-style ham, deviled ham	1 ounce
Poultry: capon, duck (domestic), goose	1 ounce
Veal: breast	1 ounce
Other protein sources: Cheese: cheddar types	1 ounce

When you are eating meats, be careful about the ways they are prepared. You may have roasted, baked, or broiled meat, poultry, and fish. When you are dining in a restaurant, trim away the excess fat and ask that gravy be omitted. Try to avoid fried, grilled, sautéed, and breaded meat, fish, and poultry. When you go out for pizza and eat half of a thirteen-inch thick-crust pizza, you had better have planned ahead, because that will cost you 7 lean-meat exchanges, along with 7½ bread, 1 milk, and 2 vegetable exchanges for a total of 1,026 calories. The better shape you are in, the more often you can enjoy such delicacies.

All the meat exchanges are based on cooked food ready to eat, with no bone or fat. It is the cooked meat, the edible portion, that is the exchange. So if you have a 4-ounce patty that weighs 3 ounces when it's cooked, it counts as 3 meat exchanges rather than the 4 you started with.

FAT EXCHANGES

A single fat exchange contains 5 grams of fat and 45 calories. This list shows the kinds and amounts of fat-containing foods to use for one fat exchange. To plan a diet low in saturated fat, select only those exchanges under "Polyunsaturated Fats."

POLYUNSATURATED FATS

Avocado†	⅛ 4-inch diam.
Margarine, soft, tub or stick*	1 teaspoon
Nuts:	
Almonds†	10 whole
Pecans†	2 large whole
Peanuts†	
Spanish	20 whole
Virginia	10 whole
Walnuts	6 small
Other nuts†	6 small
Oil, corn, cottonseed, safflower, soy, sunflower	1 teaspoon
Oil, olive†	1 teaspoon
Oil, peanut†	1 teaspoon

SATURATED FATS

Bacon fat	1 teaspoon
Bacon, crisp	1 strip

* Made with corn, cottonseed, safflower, soybean, or sunflower oil only.
† Fat content is primarily monounsaturated.

Butter	1 teaspoon
Cream, light	2 tablespoons
Cream, heavy	1 tablespoon
Cream, sour	2 tablespoons
Cream cheese	1 tablespoon
French dressing**	1 tablespoon
Italian Dressing**	1 tablespoon
Lard	1 teaspoon
Margarine, regular stick	1 teaspoon
Mayonnaise**	1 teaspoon
Salad dressing, mayonnaise- type**	2 teaspoons
Salt pork	¾-inch cube

All these fats can be enjoyed out at a restaurant, but try to avoid gravies, cream sauces, and fried foods.

** If made with corn, cottonseed, safflower, soy or sunflower oil, can be used in fat-modified diet.

Appendix II

Meal Plans and Menus for the Exercising Diabetic

Once you have mastered the exchange system, you and your doctor can design a diet that includes foods you enjoy. The "2,200 Calorie Meal Plan" below is a flexible program that might be prescribed for an exercising diabetic, and the "Sample Menu" shows how it might be used. You can even adapt your favorite recipes to your diet by replacing or eliminating high-fat, high-calorie ingredients without sacrificing flavor. Joanne Milkereit, coauthor of *The Runner's Cookbook* and consultant on the diet section of this book, has prepared a few recipes, with their exchange-value breakdowns, as examples.

2,200-CALORIE MEAL PLAN

	Breakfast	Lunch	Supper	Snack
	Number of exchanges (calories)			
Exchange				
Milk (skim)	1 (80)	1 (80)		
Vegetables		1 (25)	2 (50)	
Fruit	2 (80)	1 (40)	1 (40)	2 (80)
Bread	3 (204)	4 (272)	3 (204)	2 (136)
Meat (lean)	2 (110)	3 (165)	4 (220)	
Fat	3 (135)	3 (135)	3 (135)	
Total calories: 2,191	609	717	649	216

SAMPLE MENU*

				Exchanges		
					Vege-	Lean	
Breakfast	Milk	Fruit	Bread	table	Meat	Fat
¾ cup orange juice		1½				
2-egg mushroom-herb omelet					2	1
cooked in 1 teaspoon butter						1
2 slices toast			2			
with 1 teaspoon margarine						1
and diet jelly						
¾ cup ready-to-eat cereal			1			
1 cup skim milk	1					
Total	1	1½	3	0	2	3
Lunch						
Salad of ⅙ avocado and 1 tomato				1		1½
Pinto Burritos, using: 2 corn tortillas			2			

* Recipes included in this chapter are starred.

116

| | | Exchanges | | | |
Lunch (cont.)	Milk	Fruit	Bread	Vege-table	Lean Meat	Fat
6 tablespoons bean filling*			2			
2 tablespoons low-fat yogurt	¼					
2 teaspoons chopped onion						
3 ounces Monterey Jack cheese					3	1½
¾ cup skim milk	¾					
Melon wedge		1				
Total	1	1	4	1	3	3

* Bean filling has two bread exchanges; beef filling has ⅓ vegetable, 1 lean meat, and ½ fat exchange.

Dinner

½ cup tomato juice				1		
2 bread sticks			1			
3¾ ounces roast turkey					3¾	
½ cup mashed potato			1			
with 1½ teaspoon margarine						1½
½ cup brussels sprouts				1		
Diet cranberries						
1 peach parfait*		1½			¼	½
1 plain roll			1			
with ½ teaspoon margarine						½
Iced tea with lemon wedge						
Total	0	1½	3	2	4	2½

RECIPES

GRANOLA

Commercial granola, available in the supermarket, contains much fat and too much sugar for diabetics. This recipe contains no sugar and little fat.

2 cups uncooked oatmeal
½ cup raw wheat germ
2 tablespoons sesame seeds

¼ cup peanut butter
¾ cup raisins

Preheat oven to 325° F. In a large flat pan, combine oatmeal, wheat germ, and seeds. Place in the oven to toast for about thirty minutes, stirring every ten minutes for even browning. Over low heat, warm the peanut butter. Stir warm peanut butter into the grains while they are still warm. Stir in raisins. Cool. Store cooled granola in airtight container. You may add artificial brown sugar to serving. Makes 7 servings.

Exchange value per serving: 1½ bread, ⅓ lean meat, 1 fat, 1 fruit

"CHAMPAGNE" COCKTAIL

¼ cup chilled white grape
    juice

Squirt lemon juice
1½ cup chilled club soda

Pour chilled grape juice into a chilled champagne glass. Add lemon juice. Pour in the soda. Makes 1 serving.

Exchange value per serving: 1 fruit

PINEAPPLE-WATERCRESS COCKTAIL

1 cup unsweetened pineap-
    ple juice

1 cup fresh watercress
    sprigs

Put both ingredients into a blender. Blend well. Serve immediately. Makes 3 servings.

Exchange value per serving: 1 fruit

TROPICAL SHRIMP COCKTAIL

1 ounce shelled and de-
veined shrimp
½ cup drained pineapple
chunks

Julienne green pepper strips
Lettuce, as desired
2 tablespoons cocktail sauce

Arrange shrimp, pineapple, and green pepper on lettuce. Serve
with the cocktail sauce. Makes 1 serving.
Exchange value: 1 lean meat, 1 fruit, 1 vegetable

SAVORY CHEESE SPREAD

This cheese spread is also good as a dip with raw vegetables.

1 cup low-fat cottage cheese
2 teaspoons lemon juice
4 ounces Neufchatel cheese
5 pimiento-stuffed olives,
cut up

¼ cup chopped onion
½ teaspoon Worcestershire
sauce
½ teaspoon chili powder

Place cottage cheese and lemon juice into blender and process
until smooth. Add remaining ingredients and blend until well
combined. Makes 1½ cups.
Exchange value for ¼ cup: 1 lean meat, 1 fat

BROILED HALIBUT WITH SHRIMP SAUCE

¼ cup slivered almonds
2 tablespoons butter, melted
3 tablespoons seasoned
breadcrumbs
1 teaspoon paprika
¼ teaspoon salt
4 halibut steaks (5 ounces
each)

½ can condensed cream of
shrimp soup
¼ cup low-fat yogurt
½ teaspoon lemon rind
3 tablespoons grated Par-
mesan cheese

Heat oven to 350° F. Place almonds in a shallow pan and toast for about 15 minutes. Set aside. Turn oven to broil.

Brush some of the melted butter on a shallow broiler pan. Combine crumbs, paprika, and salt. Coat the steaks on both sides with the crumb mixture and place them on the buttered broiler pan. Drizzle remaining butter on fish. Broil four inches from the heat for about 10 minutes or until the fish flakes easily when tested with a fork.

Meanwhile, whisk together the condensed shrimp soup and the yogurt. Heat gently just to serving temperature. Whisk in the rind and the cheese.

To serve, place the steaks on a heated platter and spoon on the sauce. Sprinkle with almonds. Makes 4 servings.

Exchange value per serving: ½ bread, 4 lean meat, 3 fat

CLOSE TO BEEF STROGANOFF

Classic beef stroganoff calls for beef from the sirloin and sour cream. Those two ingredients contain too much fat. Our variation is very tasty.

1½ pounds round steak, trimmed of fat	½ cup chopped onion
2 tablespoons flour	¾ cup water
2 tablespoons oil	2 tablespoons ketchup
1 cup fresh mushrooms, sliced	1 clove garlic
	1 teaspoon salt
	¾ cup low-fat yogurt

Cut meat into strips of 1½ by 1 inch. Toss with the flour. Heat 1 tablespoon of the oil in a skillet and sauté the mushrooms and onions until the vegetables are tender. Remove vegetables from the skillet using a slotted spoon. Add the remaining oil and brown the meat over medium-high heat.

When the meat is browned, add all the remaining ingredients *except the yogurt.* Cover and simmer for 35 to 45 minutes, or until the meat is tender. Check occasionally, and add more water if necessary. Stir in the yogurt and cook only until heated through. Makes 4 servings.

Exchange value per serving: ¼ milk, 1 vegetable, 4 lean meat, 1½ fat

BEEF FILLING FOR TOSTADAS

1 pound 85 percent lean ground beef	8-ounce can tomato sauce
1 cup chopped onion	1 teaspoon chili powder
	½ teaspoon salt

Brown beef well and drain. Add chopped onions and cook for 5 minutes. Add sauce and seasonings. Reduce the heat and simmer for about 15 minutes to blend the flavors. Makes 12 servings.

Exchange value per serving: ⅓ vegetable, 1 lean meat, ½ fat

PINTO BEAN FILLING FOR BURRITOS OR TOSTADAS

½ pound dried pinto beans, cooked and drained	⅛ teaspoon powdered cumin
1½ teaspoon garlic salt	Pinch dry red pepper

Mash the beans. Mix in the seasonings. When ready to serve, heat gently in a heavy saucepan. Add a little hot water, if needed, to make the mixture smooth. Makes 2½ cups.

Exchange value for 3 tablespoons: 1 bread

SPINACH CUSTARD

Quiche is a popular dish with most people. However, the pastry is high in calories and contains a large proportion of fat. Luckily, the fillings may be prepared and baked in quiche pans or in pie plates without the pastry shell. Experiment with your favorite recipe. Reduce the baking temperature about 50° F., but bake for the same length of time.

10-ounce package frozen chopped spinach, thawed and thoroughly drained
¼ cup chopped green onion
1 tablespoon vegetable oil
3 eggs, beaten
1½ cup water

⅔ cup nonfat dry milk
½ teaspoon salt
½ teaspoon black pepper
½ teaspoon nutmeg
¾ cup grated Swiss cheese (3 ounces)

Sauté the onion for 3 to 5 minutes in the oil. Add well-drained (even squeezed) spinach, and cook for a few minutes.

Beat the eggs in a large bowl. Add water, dry milk, and seasonings. Slowly add the spinach mixture. Blend. Pour into the quiche dish or Pyrex pie plate that has been sprayed with a nonstick agent. Top with the cheese. Bake at 325° F. for 30 minutes, or until a table knife inserted into the quiche comes out clean. Makes 4 servings.

Exchange value per serving: ½ milk, ½ vegetable, 1½ lean meat, 2 fat

ZUCCHINI WITH HERBS

1 pound zucchini
1 tablespoon olive oil
Salt and pepper to taste
1 tablespoon butter
1 teaspoon chopped garlic
1 tablespoon chopped parsley

½ tablespoon chopped chives
1 teaspoon dillweed
1 teaspoon dry basil
½ teaspoon dry tarragon

Rinse zucchini and pat dry. Trim off the ends, but do not peel. Cut the zucchini into thin slices, enough to make about 6 cups. Heat the oil in a skillet. When the oil is hot, add the zucchini. Shake and toss over high heat. Add the salt and pepper. Cover.

Reduce the heat and cook for about 5 minutes. Drain in a sieve. In the same skillet, melt the butter and sauté the garlic. Then add the cooked zucchini and the herbs; toss. Serve when hot. Makes 6 servings.

Exchange value per serving: 1 vegetable, 1 fat

EGG AND POTATO BAKE

2 medium-sized potatoes, boiled and sliced	½ teaspoon salt
	½ teaspoon pepper
6 ounces thinly sliced mozzarella cheese	3 tablespoons parmesan cheese
4 eggs	1 tablespoon butter

Place the sliced potatoes in a greased shallow baking pan and place slices of mozzarella over them. Crack the eggs one at a time into a small dish, and gently ease the eggs onto the cheese. Sprinkle with salt, pepper, and Parmesan. Dot with butter. Bake in a moderately hot oven (375° F.) for about 20 minutes. Serve immediately. Makes 4 servings.

Exchange value per serving: ½ bread, 3 lean meat, 2 fat

TASTY FISH CHOWDER

2 slices bacon	1 teaspoon salt
1 cup chopped onion	¼ teaspoon pepper
16 ounces frozen fish fillets (preferably haddock), partially thawed	2 tablespoons margarine (or part bacon fat and part margarine)
1 cup chopped celery	¼ cup flour
3 small potatoes, diced	13-ounce can evaporated skim milk
2½ cups water	

In heavy saucepan, cook bacon until crisp. Drain on a paper towel. Drain and reserve fat. Add the onion to the same saucepan, and sauté until golden brown. Add the fish (cut into bite-sized pieces), celery, potatoes, water, salt, and pepper. Bring to boiling point and reduce heat. Cover and simmer 15 to 20 minutes, or until potatoes are tender.

In a small heavy saucepan, heat the margarine over low heat. Add flour and cook and stir. Gradually stir in the milk; do not dilute. Stir constantly until the white sauce is thick and bubbly. Stir white sauce into fish mixture. Crumble in the crisp bacon. Cook until thoroughly heated. Makes 6 servings.
Exchange value per serving: ½ milk, ½ bread, 1 vegetable, 3 lean meat, 1 fat

FLUFFY GRAPE GEL

A variety of simple but refreshing desserts can be made using plain gelatin and fruit juices.

1 tablespoon granulated gelatin	1½ cup unsweetened grape juice
¼ cup cold water	1 tablespoon lemon juice
½ cup boiling water	½ teaspoon lemon extract

Add gelatin to the cold water to soften. Add the boiling water. Stir to dissolve. Add the juices and extracts. Chill until nearly set, stirring every hour or so. When it is nearly set, beat with an electric mixer until very frothy. Pour into six dessert dishes, and chill until set. Makes 6 servings.
Exchange value per serving: 1 fruit

PEACH PARFAITS

An attractive dessert for a company dinner. Sugar-free strained fruits make this easy to prepare. Look for these in the baby food department.

2 ounces Neufchatel cheese
Milk
4½-ounce jar strained peaches processed without sugar
4 ripe peaches, chopped

Warm the cheese to room temperature and mash with enough milk (about 1 tablespoon) to make it smooth. Place a scant tablespoon of the peach purée in the bottom of each of four wineglasses. Top with a teaspoon of the cheese mixture. Divide evenly the chopped peaches into the glasses. Divide the remaining purée into the glass and top with the remaining cheese. Chill. Makes 4 servings.

Exchange value per serving: 1½ fruit, ¼ lean meat, ½ fat

Glossary

Adipose: Of fat, fatty.

Cholesterol: A white, waxy-looking crystalline alcohol present in human tissues. In the blood an elevated level is correlated with accelerated atherosclerosis (hardening of the arteries).

Diastole: The period of time during which the heart is filling and the blood is being ejected.

Glomerulosclerosis: Hardening of the arteries (atherosclerosis) of the kidney.

Ischemic heart disease: Heart disease due to blockage (atherosclerosis) of the arteries of the heart.

Ketones or ketone bodies: Substances with the characterizing atom group (CO) linking two hydrocarbon groups; dimethylketone (acetone) is the most important in medicine. Ketonemia refers to acetone bodies in the blood, whereas ketonuria refers to acetone substances in the urine.

Lipoproteins: A compound of protein with a fatty acid. High-density lipoprotein (HDL) are thought to guard against, and low-density lipoprotein (LDL) accelerate, atherosclerosis (hardening of the arteries).

Metabolic ketoacidosis: A metabolic state wherein ketone (acetone) bodies are being produced.

Retinopathy: Atherosclerosis (hardening of the arteries) of the eye.

Triglycerides: Fatty acids found in the blood.

Bibliography

ALLAN, F. N. "Diabetes Before and After Insulin." *Med. Hist.* 16 (1972):266–73.

ALLAN, J. W. "The relation of the pancreas to diabetes." *Lancet* 1 (1904):1343–4.

BEST, C. H. "Nineteen Hundred Twenty-One in Toronto." *Diabetes* 21 (1972): Supp. 2:385–95.

BIERMAN, E. L.; ALBRINK, M. J.; ARKY, R. A., ET AL. "Special report: Principles of nutrition and dietary recommendations for patients with diabetes mellitus." *Diabetes* 20 (1971):633–34.

BIERMAN, J., TOOHEY, B. *The Diabetic's Sports and Exercise Book.* New York: J. B. Lippincott, Co., 1977.

BJORTORP, P.; FAHLEN, M.; GRIMBY, G., ET AL. "Carbohydrate and lipid metabolism in middle-aged, physically trained men." *Metabolism* 21 (1972):1037–44.

BLACKSHEAR, P. J.; ROHDE, T. D.; PROSL, F.; BUCHWALD, H. "The implantable infusion pump: A new concept in drug delivery." *Med. Progr. Technol.* 6 (1979):149–61.

BUCHWALD, H.; ROHDE, T. D.; DORMAN, F. D.; SKAKOON, J. G.; WIGNESS, B. D.; PROSL, F. R.; TUCKER, E. M.; RUBLEIN, T. G.; BLACKSHEAR, P. J.; VARCO, R. L. "A totally implantable drug infusion device: Laboratory and clinical experience using a model with single flow rate and new design for modulated insulin infusion." *Diabetes Care* 3 (1980):351–58.

BIBLIOGRAPHY

CELSUS, A. C. *De Re Medicinae.* 3 vol. Translated by W. G. Spenser. Cambridge: Loeb Classical Library, Harvard University Press, 1935.

CRAIGHEAD, J. E. "Current views on the etiology of insulin-dependent diabetes." *New Eng. J. Med.* 299 (1978):1439–45.

CUDWORTH, A. G.; GAMBLE, D. R.; WHITE, G. B. B., ET AL. "An etiology of juvenile-onset diabetes: a prospective study." *Lancet* 1 (1977): 385–88.

DECKERT, T.; LORUP, B. "Regulation of brittle diabetes by a preplanned insulin infusion programme." *Diabetologia* 12 (1976):573–79.

DUBOS, R. "Adapting man adapting: curing, helping, consoling." *Yale J. Biol. Med.* 52 (1979):211–18.

FELIG, P.; WAHREN, J. "Fuel homeostasis in exercise." *New Eng. J. Med.* 293 (1975):1078–84.

FLETCH, A. P. "The Effect of Weight Reduction upon the Blood Pressure of Obese Hypertensives." *Quarterly J. Med.* 23 (1954): 331–45.

FLINT, M. M.; DRINKWATER, B. L.; HORVATH, S. M. "Effects of training on women's response to submaximal exercise." *Med. Sci. Sports* 6 (1974):89–94.

FLOOD, T. M. "Diet and Diabetes." *Hospital Practice* 14 (1979):61–69.

GABBAY, K. "New Directions in Diabetes." *Children's World* 4 (1977):2–17.

GENUTH, S.; MARTIN, P. "Control of hyperglycemia in adult diabetics by pulsed insulin delivery." *Diabetes* 26 (1977):571–81.

HACKETT, T. P.; CASSEM, N. H. *Exercise and the Heart.* Cardiovascular Clinics, Albert N. Best, M.D., Editor-in-Chief. Philadelphia: F. A. Davis Company, 1978.

HOLMES, O. W.; HALL, M. *Principles of the Theory and Practice of Medicine.* Boston: Little, Brown, 1939.

HUANG, S. W., MACLAREN, N. K. "Antibodies to nucleic acids in juvenile-onset diabetes. *Diabetes* 27 (1978):1105–11.

IRVINE, W. J. "Classification of idiopathic diabetes." *Lancet* 1 (1977): 638–41.

KAWATE, R.; MIYANISKI, M.; NISHIMOTO, Y. "Prevalence and mortality of diabetes mellitus in Japanese in Hawaii and Japan." In BABA, S., ET AL., "Diabetes Mellitus in Asia." *Amsterdam Exerpta Medica* (1976).

KOIVISTO, V. A; FELIG, P: "Effects of leg exercise on insulin absorption in diabetic patients." *New Eng. J. Med.* 298 (1978):79–83.

KUZUYA, T.; IRIE, M.; NILA, Y. "Glucose intolerance among Japanese professional sumo-wrestlers." In BABA, S., ET AL., "Diabetes mellitus in Asia." *Amsterdam Exerpta Medica* (1976).

LAWRENCE, R. D. "The effect of exercise on insulin in diabetes." *Br. Med. J.* 1 (1926):648–50.

LIKE, A. A.; APPEL, M. C.; WILLIAMS, R. M.; ROSSINI, A. A. "Streptozotocin-induced pancreatic insulinitis in mice. Morphologic and physiologic studies." *Lab. Invest.* 38:4 (1978):470–86.

LIV, N., CURETON, T. K., JR. "Effects of training on maximal oxygen intake of middle-aged women." *Amer. Corr. Ther. J.* 29 (1975):56–61.

MACLEOD, J. J. R. "History of the Researches Leading to the Discovery of Insulin." *Bull. Hist. of Med.* 52 (1978):295–312.

MAEHLUM, S. "Muscular exercise and metabolism in male juvenile diabetes. II Glucose tolerance after exercise." *Scand. J. Clin. Lab. Invest.* 32 (1973):145–53.

MAJOR, R. H. *Classic Descriptions of Disease*, 3rd ed. Oxford: Blackwell Scientific Publications, 1948.

MATAS, A. J.; SUTHERLAND, D. E. R.; NAJARIAN, J. S. "Current status of islet and pancreas transplantation in diabetes." *Diabetes* 25 (1976):785–95.

NABARRO, J. D.; MUSTAFFA, B. E.; MORRIS, D. V., ET AL. "Insulin deficient diabetes: contrasts with other endocrine deficiencies." *Diabetologia* 16 (1979):5–12.

NOTKINS, A. L. "The cause of diabetes." *Scientific American* 241 (1979):62–73.

PEDERSEN, O.; HENNING, B. N.; HEDING, L. "Increased insulin receptors after exercise in patients with insulin-dependent diabetes mellitus." *New Eng. J. Med.* 302 (1980):886–91.

PICKUP, J. C.; KEEN, H.; PARSON, J. A.; ALBERTI, K. G. M. M. "Continuous subcutaneous insulin infusion: An approach to achieving normoglycaemia." *Br. Med. J.* 1 (1978):204–7.

PONIKOWSKA, I. "Effect of graded physical exercise on blood sugar level in healthy subjects and diabetics." *Pol. Tyg. Lek.* 27 (1972):1961–63.

PURETT, E. D. R., MAEHLUM, S. "Muscular exercise and metabolism in male juvenile diabetics." *Scand. J. Clin. Lab. Invest.* 32 (1973):139–47.

PYKE, D. A., NELSON, P. G. "Diabetes mellitus in identical twins." In *The Genetics of Diabetes Mellitus,* edited by W. Creutzfeldt, J. Kobberling, J. V. Neel, pp. 194–202. Berlin: Springer-Verlag, 1976.

BIBLIOGRAPHY

RUSSELL, P. S.; COSIMI, A. B. "Transplantation." *New Eng. J. Med.* 301 (1979):470-79.

Saint Louis Park Medical Center Research Foundation Newsletter 1 (1980):1.

SCHAFER, E. A. In *The Endocrine Organs,* p. 128. London: Longmans, 1916.

SERVICE, F. J. "Normalization of plasma glucose of unstable diabetics: studies under ambulatory, fed conditions with pumped intravenous insulin." *J. Lab. Clin. Med.* 91 (1978):480-89.

SLAMA, G.; HAUTECOUVERTURE, M.; ASSAN, R; TCHOBROUTSKY, G. "One to five days of continuous intravenous insulin infusion in seven diabetic patients." *Diabetes* 23: (1974):732-38.

SOMAN, V. R.; KOIVISTO, V. A.; DEIBERT, D.; FELIG, P.; DEFRANZO, R. A. "Increased insulin sensitivity and insulin binding to monocytes after physical training." *New Eng. J. Med.* 301 (1979):1200-1204.

TAMBORLANE, M. V.; SHERWIN, R. S.; GENOL, M.; FELIG, P. "Reduction to normal of plasma glucose in juvenile diabetes by subcutaneous administration of insulin with a portable infusion pump." *New Eng. J. Med.* 300 (1979):573-78.

TRUSWELL, A. S., MANN, J. I. "Epidemiology of serum lipids in Southern Africa." *Atherosclerosis* 16 (1972):15-29.

VAN HANDEL, P. J.; COSTILL, D. L.; GETCHELL, I. H. "Central circulatory adaptations to physical training." *Res. Q. Am. Assoc. Health Phys. Ed.* 47 (1976):815-23.

WAHREN, J.; FELIG, P.; AHLBORG, G, ET AL. "Glucose metabolism during leg exercise in man." *J. Clin. Invest.* 50 (1971):2715-25.

―――. "Glucose and free fatty acid utilization in exercise studies in normal and diabetic man." *Israel J. Med. Sci.* 11 (1975):551-59.

WEST, K. M. "Epidemiologic evidence linking nutritional factors to the prevalence and manifestation of diabetes." *Diabetol. Lat.* 9 (1972):405-28.

―――. "Diet therapy of diabetes: An analysis of failure." *Ann. Intern. Med.* 79 (1973):425-34.

―――. "Diabetes in American Indians and other native populations of the new world." *Diabetes* 23 (1974):841-55.

―――. "Epidemiologic observations on thirteen populations of Asia and the Western hemisphere." Proceedings of VIII International Sugar Research Foundation, edited by S. S. Hillebrand, pp. 33-43, 1974.

―――. "Prevention and therapy of diabetes mellitus." *Nutr. Rev.* 33:193-98.

―――. "Diet and diabetes." *Postgraduate Medicine* 60 (1976):209–16.

―――; KALBFLEISCH, J. M. "Diabetes in Central America." *Diabetes* 19 (1970):656–68.

―――. "Influence of nutritional factors on prevalence of diabetes." *Diabetes* 20 (1971):99–108.

Index